GIVING
from the HEART

Susan P. Byrnes, R.N.

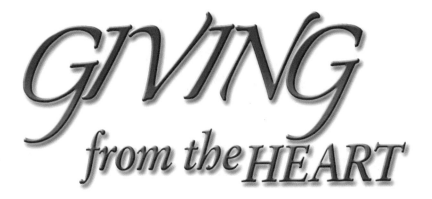

Megan,

Live Well,

Susan

GIVING from the HEART
A true story of how one woman's tragedy inspired a community.
By Susan P. Byrnes R.N.

Published by:
Susan P. Byrnes, R.N., Founder
Susan P. Byrnes Health Education Center
515 South George Street
York, PA 17401

Orders:
info@byrneshec.com
www.byrneshec.com

Unattributed quotations are by Susan Byrnes.

ISBN- 10   0-9794535-9-3
ISBN- 13   978-0-9794535-9-5

First Printing 2007

Printed in the United States of America

Library of Congress Control Number: 200790232

Contents

In memory of our beloved Mom-Mom

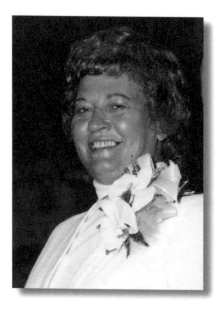

Gratitude

I wrote GIVING from the HEART to thank my community for believing in my dream of a health education center and to inspire you, the reader, to love yourself enough to take charge of your health, put your passion into action and make a difference in your community.

My heartfelt gratitude to all the volunteers; board and staff, past and present, who have given generously of their time, dedication and money to ensure the success of OUR Health Education Center.

To my "angels", you have a special place in my heart.

To Chuck Preston, Creative Director, Charles Design Group, for your in-kind donation of expertise with my beautiful book cover, layout and format, my gratitude.

To my skillful editor, Vicky, who asked probing questions, organized my thoughts and created a story far better than I could have achieved on my own. Thank you from the bottom of my heart.

I am deeply grateful for the love and encouragement from my Mother and Dad (Daddy), extended family and dear friends.

I love you, Katie, Kristy and Nate, and Dan! I am humbled by the love and joy that you bring into my life.

To Randy, my husband of 1750 weeks, (as of 3/24/07) my in-house editor and entrepreneurial mentor, thank you for your love, hugs and humor that nourishes and sustains me.

My life has been deeply blessed by the people who have been part of my journey of developing a health education center for my hometown of York, PA.

Live WELL   Susan P. Byrnes, R.N.

Thoughts On Charitable Giving

When it comes to giving, it seems to me there are, generally speaking, two kinds of givers: those who give willingly, generously and frequently, and others who give grudgingly, sparingly and seldom.

I think we would agree that the kind of giver one is has little to do with financial or social status. There are those who are remarkably generous, even though for them giving is a real financial sacrifice. By contrast, some among the relatively wealthy have yet to discover the spiritual rewards true generosity can bring.

Regardless of their station in life, many have made giving almost as natural a part of their existence as eating and sleeping. For those fortunate people, giving from the heart (as Susie would say), is a time of joy and uplift. For others, the act of giving, if they do it at all, is a time of discomfort, concern and even distress. Consequently, a gift brings little if any pleasure. They truly do not know what they are missing.

John D. Rockefeller, Jr. has suggested that we "Think of giving not as a duty but as a privilege." One need not have the wherewithal of a Rockefeller to relate to that sentiment, although, I'm not sure I ever viewed the act of giving in quite that sense. Rather, I have always considered myself fortunate to be a donor, even in the early days when my young-adult resources were decidedly limited. It's worth remembering that "a gift gives twice"; once to the recipient, and second, to the giver. That has, indeed, been my experience.

As I look back over the years on the projects I have had the opportunity to support, none stands out more memorably than Susie Byrnes' dream of a center for health education. Her passion for the project was in itself totally convincing. But even beyond her emotional commitment, she had a plan that was seriously conceived and meticulously thought out. Thanks to her own special determination, skill and sincere persuasiveness, she convinced a skeptical community of the worth of her vision. Today, a hugely successful enterprise known as the Susan P. Byrnes Health Education Center educates thousands of persons each year, primarily youngsters, on the importance of a healthy lifestyle. It stands as a tribute to one unique young lady's determination, foresight, wisdom, and passion.

LJA, Jr. 11/29/06

Mr. Louis J. Appell, Jr, community leader, former board member of the Susan P. Byrnes Health Education Center

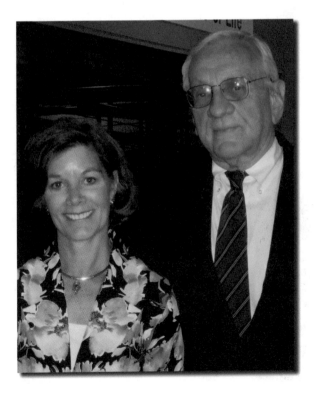

1

Conception

The myriad of machines in the Intensive Care Unit were barely keeping her alive. *Mom-Mom* was resting in bed number ten. Despite all the heaving sounds emanating from the life-support systems, we knew the prognosis was not good. Lori, my sister-in-law and I, had brought a gift from her six grandchildren. We waited in anticipation as she read the crayoned Valentine banner "We Love You, Mom-Mom, Please Get Well."

Mom-Mom Byrnes' eyes brimmed with tears. Her loss of words, muffled by the endoscope tube taped in her mouth supplying oxygen to her lungs, prevented even a smile. It was only yesterday the doctor had gently suggested she needed to get her life in order. It was being measured in tiny increments.

Mom-Mom died twelve hours later at 3:45 A.M. on Monday, February 15, 1988.

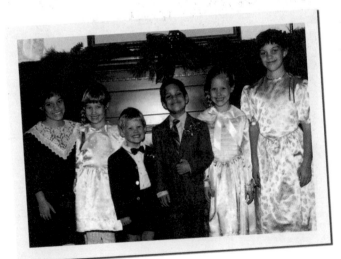

Kristy, 8, Shannon, 5, Kevin, 3, Danny, 7, Erin, 7, Katie, 10
The Grandchildren

Conception

The day after his 60 yr. old grandmother's death, I comforted my son, Danny, in my arms. He asked me why Mom-Mom had died. I explained that for many years she had smoked cigarettes that hurt her lungs and the 'special drinks' she liked caused her liver to get sick. With tears pooling in his big blue eyes and all the innocence of his seven years Danny simply asked, "If Mom-Mom loved me why did she continue to smoke and drink?"

I cried… tears of anger and intense sadness.

My anger arose because I felt as a nurse I had failed my mother-in-law by not inspiring her to make healthy choices; my sadness because our family had lost our beloved Mom-Mom. Our children, nieces and nephew would never share their confirmations, graduations or weddings with their fun-loving Mom-Mom. They would never be able to tell her about their lives and receive the unconditional love and caring that Mom-Mom gave so well. Yvonne Byrnes was my Mother-in-LOVE and the beloved Mom-Mom to my three precious little ones.

In the beginning of my relationship with her son, Randy, Mrs. Byrnes was the protective mother of her eldest "perfect" child. (Randy's facetious description of himself to his three children). From the time I was fifteen, Mrs. Byrnes ("Yok" to family and friends) had been an intimate part of my life. (In 1972, after six years of dating, Randy and I were deeply in love, (well, I knew that I was, he wasn't so sure.) We had spent the last three years sharing a long distance relationship and I wanted us to live in the same town. During another teary good-bye prior to Randy's senior year, at the University of Dayton, we decided that I would move to Ohio. We wanted to see if we truly were marriage material. I would get a roommate, Randy already had two.

Sharing this news with my parents and Randy's parents was quite controversial, even in the time of 'peace and love.' My mother and I were in total disagreement about my decision and Mrs. Byrnes called my mother to say "If she were my daughter she would not be moving to Dayton." Randy was going to be the first Byrnes/Button to graduate from college and Mrs. Byrnes didn't want any hiccups (if you know what I mean). But I was 21, had lived on my own for two years and wanted to be with Randy. I made the trek to Ohio and began to work nights at Miami Valley Hospital Emergency Department. Randy continued his college lifestyle with me now an integral part of his day. He would drive me to work at 11P.M. and return with a warm car at 7:30 A.M. What a guy! We were engaged and married within 11 months.

Mrs. Byrnes was the consummate 1950's mother who loved her children and devoted herself to them. She, and her husband, raised Randy, Lori and Mike in a small neighborhood where most moms were at home. She went to work for additional family income when her youngest entered grade school. The family's social life was getting together with life-long friends who

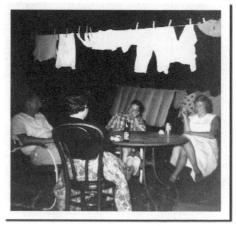

Friends from work, Jim and Yok Byrnes

worked at Caterpillar Tractor (Randy's father's employer); many of them from their hometown, Peoria IL. This 50's generation had grown up with the liberal use of tobacco, beer and hard liquor. Everybody did it. No one even suspected how deadly tobacco and alcohol were to the mind and body. These social habits were a fundamental part of the lifestyle. Movies with stars like John Wayne, Katharine Hepburn and Spencer Tracy, and a patronizing government had anesthetized an entire generation to the usage of self-inflicted poisons.

Upbeat and outgoing, Mrs. Byrnes quickly became endeared to me; as my married love with her son grew so did my love for her. Every other week-end, (my week-end off from the emergency department) Randy and I would be invited for a home-cooked meal. An added benefit was free use of the washer and dryer. When we moved to a small home in Mount Wolf, PA, Mr. and Mrs. Byrnes assisted with indoor painting, building a picnic table and furnishing the nursery. Combined family gatherings of the Byrnes and Petron (my family) households often ended in our basement in hotly contested ping-pong rallies. We were evolving into a family. Mrs. Byrnes became Yok and Yok became our children's beloved Mom-Mom.

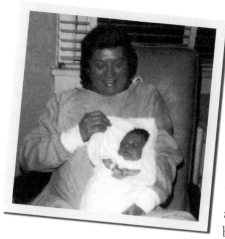

In January, 1978, our first daughter Katie was born. I had experienced several false labor starts during one of Pennsylvania's worst blizzards and I spent many nights at my in-law's home so I could be closer to the hospital. Following Katie's birth Mom-Mom became my #1 babysitter. She loved holding and talking with our beautiful blue-eyed baby. A favorite spot for these activities was on top of

Mom-Mom and Katie (first grandchild)

the portable dishwasher that was cushioned by Katie's cross-stitched blanket from Mom-Mom. This allowed Randy and me some alone time and low and behold sixteen months to the date of Katie's birth, our brown-eyed Kristy arrived. Mom-Mom rose to the challenge of helping me with our two beautiful girls and sixteen months later, she was thrilled when Daniel James completed our young family; three children under three (breast feeding is NOT a form of birth control). These precious little ones exuded love for their Mom-Mom and she responded to this love with enthusiasm and responsibility. She tempered her drinking and never smoked when she was with them. I truly depended on her support and assistance. With her dedication, love and babysitting, I was able to juggle the demands of three children and a husband's busy schedule, work part-time in the Emergency Department and be President of Young Women's Club, an organization that raises money to help children and the arts. By this time, Mom-Mom was retired and operated as my primary support system. My own mother still had children at home and was working full-time which limited her availability.

Yet, our love and devotion was not enough to inspire Yvonne to change her unhealthy habits. For ten years, Randy and I sadly watched her health deteriorate. Then in October of 1987, I noticed signs that were quite disturbing: swelling of her legs and yellowing of her sclera, the white part of her eyes. As a nurse, I knew that these could be indications of liver failure. When I mentioned my concern to her she stated that she was tired from her recent trip to Peoria, IL. She had attended her high school reunion and visited with family and friends. (Later, I wondered if she knew that she was very ill and this was a good-bye trip.)

Shortly after this conversation, Randy's brother, Mike, became engaged. Randy and I agreed to have the December wedding in our home. Lori, Randy's and Mike's sister, and I catered this festive celebration for sixty friends and relatives. Pictures were taken with many smiling faces. Little did we realize that this would be the last picture of Mom-Mom and Pop-Pop together.

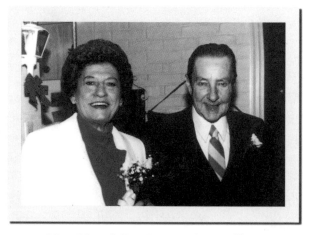

Mom-Mom & Pop-Pop at Mike's wedding

December, 1987

Six weeks later, January 26, 1988, Mom-Mom collapsed at home in the hallway leading from her bedroom and was rushed to the hospital in a hepatic coma. She spent three weeks in and out of Intensive Care. She never got to say good-bye to her six precious grandchildren.

During the painful days following her funeral, I could not shake overwhelming feelings of helplessness, frustration and anger. Adding to my personal grief, I began to reflect upon the hundreds of times that I was professionally faced with patients' unhealthy choices that had resulted in their emergency visits. One memorable admission kept coming into my mind.

It had been a hectic eight hours in the Emergency Department. No time for a dinner break. My duties as a staff nurse included supervision of Rooms 11 and 12 in the Cardiac Division. Near 8:00 P.M., Springettsbury Ambulance radioed that they had a 53 year-old male with crushing chest pain, nausea and shortness of breath. I went to Room 11 and prepared for our incoming MI (myocardial infarction) patient.

As we pulled Mr. Martin from the ambulance litter to our bed, I tried to reassure him that we would ease his chest pain and shortness of breath. In my head and heart, I knew he was gravely ill. He was sweating profusely; his breath was rapid, shallow and gurgled. An EKG, blood tests and chest X-ray confirmed our clinical diagnosis that he was having a massive heart attack and his lungs were filling with fluid. We worked for two strenuous hours. Mr. Martin was pronounced dead at 10:08 P.M.

Dr. Jansen and I slowly walked to the Emergency Department's private waiting room. I held Mrs. Martin and told her how hard we had worked to save her husband, but my heart was aching because I knew that if Mr. Martin had been fifty pounds lighter, if he had not been a smoker for many years, he could still be alive.

That night, driving home, I cried. I cried for Mom-Mom. I cried for Mrs. Martin and her family. Why did people over-eat, over-drink, smoke and not get exercise? Did people know how detrimental these habits are to their health? If they knew, would they find a way to make healthy choices for themselves and their families?

Mom-Mom's and Mr. Martin's deaths led to a series of personal actions that would change my life forever. I decided I was tired of trying to restore health to bodies ravaged with disease that, in many cases, could have been prevented. I quit my job as an Emergency Department nurse. I made a new life goal; keeping people well. When people ended up in the Emergency Department it was too late for many of them. I was determined to reach people before it was too late.

I remembered that in June, 1987, on a family vacation to Peoria, IL, I had viewed a video of a health education center that was being built through the efforts of the Junior League. As I reflected on this concept of health education taught in dramatic teaching theaters I became more and more excited. The answer to all of my questions was IN MOM-MOM'S HOMETOWN.

I decided I was going to create a health education center in my own hometown of York, Pennsylvania. I shared my idea with my entrepreneurial husband. Randy had built an employment business from three people to fifty. It became the largest custom staffing organization in the region. He knew that it took grueling hours and years of dedication to build a business from scratch... let alone a dream for a not-for-profit. He put his arms around me and said "Katie, Kristy and Danny are only 10, 8 and 7. Are you sure you want to do this? Do you have any idea how much work and energy will be involved?" I had no clue. He did.

I told him that I had to do this to honor his mother. If I can keep one family from grieving about the loss of a loved one due to unhealthy choices it would be worth my time and energy.

I began by keeping a red notebook with journal notes from every call that I made, to people who were building health education centers across the country, and to people in my community who I wanted to support my dream.

The first entry was March, 1988.

At this time, there were only ten health education centers in the U.S. I began to visit these organizations speaking with the board members and executive directors, making copious notes. I tried to limit the time away from my young family, but I quickly realized that Randy was correct; my dream of creating a health education center was going to take years.

I drove to Easton, PA to visit the Weller Health Education Center. When I saw the exhibits, enthusiastic educators and the impact of the Substance Abuse education on the fifty visiting fourth graders, my heart filled with joy. I knew these dynamic health education lessons that I had witnessed would motivate little ones to make healthy choices perhaps for the rest of their lives. The three hour ride home to York flew by. Adrenaline was pulsing through my veins and arteries. In my mind I began to plan how I would begin to build a health education center.

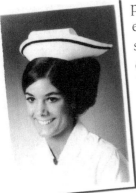

As a nurse, I thought that one of my first prospect meetings should be with my former employer, the largest hospital in the area. After several phone calls and a meeting with employees in the Health Promotion Department, it became abundantly clear that the hospital's mission of treating disease fell short of my mission... I wanted to educate people about their bodies and inspire them to make healthy choices. (Keep in mind, this was 1988, health promotion was not yet a national priority... will it ever be???)

1971 Great nurse's cap...

That spring and summer I was very involved in volunteering at a decorator's showhouse project, a fund-raiser led by the Young Women's Club of York. The duties and pleasures of being a mom for three young children in the summertime brought a period of joy and togetherness to our growing family. Health education center meetings were put on hold until school resumed.

September 22, 1988, I returned to Peoria, IL, (Mom-Mom's birthplace) and met with Patty Bash, a Junior League member, who was spearheading the creation of their health education center. We hit it off immediately and saw eye-to-eye (we are both five feet tall) on our passion for prevention. Patty was the President of the Center's Board of Directors and she graciously offered to let me attend and observe their next meeting. I listened attentively as the committee members reported on their progress. After copying Patty's entire historical notebook, I made prints of her slideshow.

The next day, I traveled to the Robert Crown Health Education Center in Hinsdale, IL. I again took copious notes. I had little working knowledge of cameras and computers. This minute but dedicated group of health education leaders was very helpful. They were on a special journey. I was about to join their mission. Later that day, I met Richard Rush in his Chicago Studios. Rush Studios was the lone exhibit maker for all ten operational health education centers in the country. He gave me a pamphlet, "How to Build Your Health Education Center." I returned to York and immediately became overwhelmed with how much there was to do but... "The journey of a thousand miles begins with a single step." (Lao-tzu, Chinese Philosopher)

On October 14, 1988, I conducted the first presentation for the Health Education Center in York in my home. The meeting was to begin at 7:30 P.M. At 7:00 P.M., I had a towel wrapped around my head and Randy was supervising a boisterous bath and story time for our three children. With wet hair and thirty minutes to spare, I franticly maneuvered through the house looking for a three-pronged plug for my slide projector. My lack of technology skills was obvious - not good for one who wants to create a high-tech health education center, I thought.

The first obligatory attendants to my presentation were my dentist, doctor, accountant and a few close friends. The event was a success despite my harried preparations. The group thought the slide show impressive and inspiring but questioned the affordability of a health education center in York. Their well meaning and insightful questions indicated just how much needed to be done:

- Where will it be located?
- How many students will it hold?
- How will the schools pay for this?
- Who will build these displays?
- Can our community support another not-for-profit?
- Why aren't the hospitals providing health education?

Everyone said it was a good idea... but no one volunteered to help. I knew in my heart that somehow I had to make my dream happen.

Several weeks later, my first angel appeared, one with accounting skills, Jim Bergdoll. His parents had both been healthcare professionals; his father a highly regarded surgeon, his mother a hard-working nurse. They had dedicated many years to the health of families in our community. While enjoying an

Oktoberfest at his rural home, Jim shared with me that in honor of his parents he would become a board member. The HEC's first board member! (After 18 years, Jim is still our Finance Chair) With Jim's support and business network, I began to surround myself with people who possessed the professional assets to offset my weaknesses: finance, business and legal matters were first on the list.

January, 1989, I conducted my first board meeting. Present were five dedicated people; my children's elementary school principal, Jim, our accountant, an attorney referred by Jim, a banker, our insurance representative and me. I affectionately referred to them as the "fab five." We met every month and I would report on my progress of creating awareness through my phone calls and presentations.

Two months later, March, 1989, The IRS declared us to be an official not-for-profit 501(c)(3) organization. The Central Pennsylvania Health Education Center (HEC) was "conceived". Oh my, what had I done? I was thrilled and frightened all in the same moment. I was a nurse, not a business person. How do I build a not-for-profit? How much money would I need? How could I raise that money? Would anyone even come?

I prayed and prayed that I was using my gifts from God the way that He wanted. I took long walks and asked for a sign that God really wanted me to give my time and energy to building a health education center. God responded. Good things began to happen.

With the official not-for-profit status I began to unleash my fund raising talents on the community. The Young Women's Club was the first to approve my grant request. With their $500 donation, I rented a bus and filled it with members of the Medical Allicance and Young Women's Club.

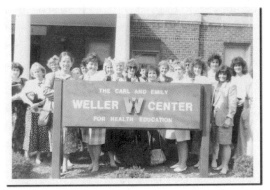

My first converts

We traveled two plus hours to the Weller Health Education Center in Easton, PA. (I had observed my very first health education program there one year earlier) This was a very important litmus test for the potential affirmation of a health education center in our community. It was a resounding success.

The bus ride home was filled with animated conversations and a wonderful enthusiasm to move this project forward. The first real community-wide support for a York HEC had been established. I felt tingly and fluttering sensations all over my body. Could this be the initial moment that I experienced the "life" ("quickening" in medical terms) of the health education center?

My husband Randy was my behind- the-scenes support net. His constant encouragement to "smile and dial" and "meet and greet" buffeted my crusade of spreading the word. Daily calls to him of disappointments and joys became the norm. At night, we would review strategy and talk and talk.

It was exhilarating and exhausting.

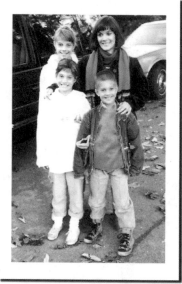

Katie and me in the back, Kristy and Dan

I did not know that the "pregnancy" would last seven years and be filled with moments of tremendous self-doubt, extreme fatigue and motherly guilt.

In the fall of 1989, I was eighteen months into my crusade when something happened that really shook me up. One Sunday morning, our 10 yr. old daughter Kristy returned from a birthday sleepover in acute respiratory distress. She had asthma and had been exposed to secondhand smoke when the children went bowling as part of the birthday festivities. I drove quickly to the Emergency Department. She received immediate attention; a needle was inserted into a vein in her left hand and intravenous fluids began to drip into her circulatory system, then, the drug, epinephrine, was injected into her right deltoid muscle of her upper arm. She was in a state of status asthmaticus... the smallest tubes in her lungs were in spasm and filled with mucous...her tissues were not getting enough oxygen. The fluids and medicine began to work and the wheezing in her lungs began to subside a little. She was admitted to the Pediatric floor and I slept with her for two nights as steroids and fluids were infused into her little body. It was one of the scariest times of my life.

Tuesday morning I gently explained that I had an important meeting for the health education center at Dad's office and I would only be gone for two hours. I left my daughter's hospital room to chair a Board meeting for the nascent HEC at which only two Board members attended.

As I drove back to the hospital I cried and told God that this was too difficult. I was leaving my sick child in a hospital to chair a meeting about a concept that was of no interest to anyone but me... I almost gave up my dream.

Randy encouraged me to take a few days off and devote them to getting Kristy well.

I did.

My recovery coincided with hers.

2

Embryo

Just as the embryonic sac cushions and protects a growing fetus, my hometown of York, Pennsylvania, surrounded and supported me during the development of my seven-year dream come true.

Beautiful rolling hills in the Susquehanna River Valley; the professed First Capital of the United States; home to a hard-working agricultural and manufacturing community; generous givers; incorporated in 1741; these are the touchstones of my hometown.

I grew up on Cherry St. in Spry, just south of the city. One of seven children, we were the '50's poster family (except maybe the seven children part). Our house had two bedrooms, one full bathroom and a powder room...eventually; the basement was converted into three more bedrooms. On your birthday you were treated like a Queen/King for the day; no chores, your favorite dinner and dessert and a scavenger hunt to find your presents. (The number of clues was determined by the number of birthdays that you were celebrating).

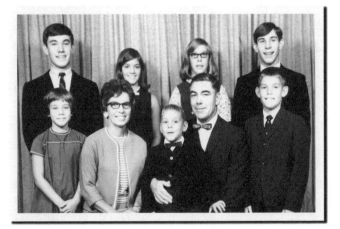

Petron family, 1967 I'm second from left in back row

Embryo

My father was a South Philadelphia boy whose father had changed his surname from Petroccione to Petron to offset the bigotry of the times in 1920. My dad fought in WWII; returned to finish college; met his future wife; helped raise seven children and spent forty years of his life selling business forms. Today, at 84 years old, he works three days a week part-time and completes math puzzles in his head before we can retrieve a pencil to write down the problem.

My German-born mother left her hometown of Bochum and set sail from Antwep, Belgium, on the Belgenland. On July 28, 1928, at the age of five, she arrived in the New York Harbor. Despite having to learn English, she breezed through public school, even skipping a grade. She was Valedictorian of her high school class and received as a reward a subscription to Readers Digest. However, she was denied the opportunity to attend college classes because she could not afford the tuition. She became a waitress at Penn State's Corner Room in State College, PA, a local landmark, and audited classes. In February, 1947 my Dad asked to copy her notes from their sociology class. They married five months later. She became the stay-at-home mother who, among other innumerable responsibilities, sold holiday cards to provide Christmas gifts for her seven children. As further evidence of the stock from which I come, my mother at the age of 57 ran for public office as the Township Tax Collector, won and held the position for the next twelve years. In addition, she has served as a Republican Committee Woman in York Township for the last four decades.

I expound on my parents' backgrounds because you can learn a great deal about someone by knowing who was shaping the first eighteen years of their lives. Mine were formed by two church-going, hard-working, self-reliant people who struggled mightily to provide for the safety and security of their large family. I am a small mirror of their character.

My parents were, and continue to be, very involved in their community. This lesson was brought home to me as a junior in high school when, at the dinner table on a weekday, my father asked what I was doing downtown in the middle of the day. Flabbergasted, I asked how he knew such a thing. He just grinned and said "York is a small town. I have spies everywhere."

Little did I know that this same small town with 'spies everywhere' would someday be the network of business leaders and community philanthropists who would make the Health Education Center blossom into existence.

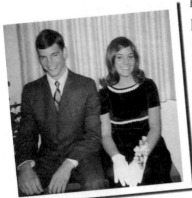

Randy and Susie
Homecoming, 1966

Randy and I met at an eighth grade party. We went to different grade schools but one of my girlfriends had just moved from Randy's grade school to mine and she had a party for her St. Pat's and St. Joe's school friends. I observed this handsome athlete from afar. And then we met again at the local catholic high school. We were both in the common experiences of puppy love... with other people. In fact, I was head over heals in love with one of his close friends. This 'love affair' was terminated when the five foot Prefect of Discipline, Sister Marie Aquin, called my beau's father and told him, that his son was spending too much time with Susan Petron and that she would jeopardize his chances for becoming President of the student body - in three years. Several months after this traumatic ending to my first love, Randy became my true high school sweetheart at the age of fifteen. (Three years later he was elected VP of the school, and my "first love" lost the election). We were married Labor Day weekend of 1973.

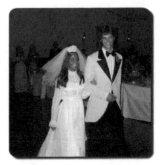

Wedding Day, 9/1/73

Randy is my knight in shining armor, my in-house editor and my best friend of 40 years. Together, we have accomplished more than either of us would have dreamed possible on our own. Randy's level head and entrepreneurial expertise complements my compassionate social action. His success in business provided financial security for our family and my ever expanding universe as a small town philanthropist. It also opened doors for me.

Randy's business connections enabled me to meet with established families and community leaders. The Health Education Center became a recipient of the generosity of hundreds of individuals' and corporations' time, talent and treasures.

Over the next two years, I made 225 presentations. Individuals, groups and clubs were my targets, no one was safe; Rotary, Sertoma, Junior League, Seroptimists and Optimists Clubs; school superintendents and principals; business and healthcare professionals. I encountered every response from indifference to ovations.

At one presentation to a group of all male high school principals I was scheduled next to last on the agenda. Following the first priority, a thorough review of the high school football standings and who was beating whom, I

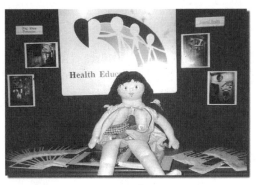

Organ Annie, a prop for presentations,
With removable organs.

was introduced to reserved applause and an audience with a total lack of interest in my presentation on the benefits of health education in our schools. This was my future customer base?

Not Good.

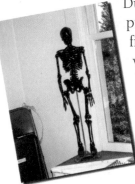

During another presentation to a group of professional healthcare givers I was allocated fifteen minutes at 10:00 P.M. during their weekly staff meeting. I made my plea for the benefits of prevention; how the HEC would be a tremendous asset to our community and the important role that they could have in leading this effort. The response - absolute silence; not a question, not a word - nothing.

I made more presentations than
Charlie Chan's bone count: 206

It was another long ride home. I drove while thinking about the fact that I had given up bedtime rituals with my three little ones to travel through a driving rain storm for 25 minutes to make this presentation to a group of HEALTHCARE PROFESSIONALS who didn't care about prevention. My physical and emotional exhaustion was deepening. My children were sound asleep, once again when I got home. I went into Randy's arms and cried.

There is obviously an upside to this story or I wouldn't be writing and you wouldn't be reading. As word spread and my presentations continued, a number of the business and healthcare leaders began to take notice. A self-made insurance executive, who had built a national company from very humble beginnings, allowed me the use of his airplane to transport potential supporters and givers to visit health education centers around the country. A local printing business produced our first brochure for free and a number of other business executives joined my dream by sharing their expertise and money as well as lending their key managers to serve on our board.

Momentum was building. My passion and persistence were fueling a fire of excitement. But supporters and board members were not in agreement on the most significant decision; the location and size of the yet-to-be-born health education center.

In a memorable meeting held in the board room of a locally-based, international company Jim Bergdoll and I were told by an important group of community executives that they had successfully located a site for me; two rooms on the second floor of an agricultural museum. The students were going to have to climb, run, and possibly fall down twenty narrow steps. I was not interested. Clearly, we had different visions. I politely declined their offer that apparently (by the looks and deafening silence) was not done very often. After the meeting Jim shared with me that he could feel the tension in the room when I gave my quick response of immediate dismissal and rejection to the leaders of our community. This surprised me. I guess being naive has its advantages; I never sensed their power and disappointment. Nevertheless, the meeting proved to be a valuable learning point for all parties as I began to realize that the person with the money makes the rules and my fellow community leaders became aware that I was what was later referred to as "intractable" in my passion to create the finest HEC in the country. There may have been additional adjectives used but I know of only this one.

In a subsequent meeting with a bank President and a few other board members, we were reviewing the plusses and minuses of a long list of potential sites. After a particularly exasperating hour of debating site after site that I rejected, he said "What is it you want?" to which I replied "About three million dollars from that vault behind you."

He got a good laugh, we got our desired site. (more on the site in the Seven Year Pregnancy chapter)

The people of York and South Central PA are hard-working, conservative and generous. Where else could a petite nurse from Spry, with a dream to keep people healthy, secure almost three million dollars in gifts and pledges through the efforts of volunteers, local businesses and community philanthropists?

During the past nineteen years my life has been deeply enriched by thousands of local residents who have given their time, talents and treasures to create a leading resource for innovative, high-quality and effective health education.

When I give tours I tell visitors that if I had been born in another town, the Byrnes Health Education Center would not exist. No matter where I may roam, York will always be my home!

The conception of the Health Education Center, sometimes similar to conception in life, was the easy and fun part. It only took eighteen months. The pregnancy proved to be much longer …it took almost seven years…four times longer then the gestation period of an elephant!

3

Seven Year Pregnancy

Pregnancy can bring about extreme changes in the female body: nausea, vomiting, heartburn, shortness of breath, weight gain, backache and little time, energy or desire for intimacy. Can you imagine the symptoms from a seven year pregnancy? I can attest to the fact that I experienced each of the above maladies to the 7th degree.

In 1991, as I entered the third year of my health education pregnancy, I recognized two things: first, my dream was expanding in scope and scale and I needed additional expertise and guidance, much like the expectant mother chooses her delivery team; second, I was

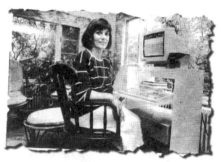

My home office (see how tired I look)

outgrowing my small office just as a mother outgrows her "normal clothes". When I first embarked on this journey, I felt secure in operating from our home office surrounded by my family and our serene five acres of trees and beautiful flower gardens. The huge oak tree and red jungle gym, where my little ones used to climb and play was visible from my desk and the sight of those fixtures gave me peace in times of chaos. But my vision for creating the premier regional resource for health education entailed a massive amount of paper work that overwhelmed my 10'x10' enclosed porch office. It was time to take our family computer and filing cabinet to new accommodations.

I also knew that I needed more time and more administrative

know-how. For several months, Pam, a mother with a young son, provided a welcome relief through her 10 hours of work with me each week. My husband's temporary services business hired and paid her salary. Pam spent her time scheduling my appointments and mailing informational packets. As a sign of my appreciation to the people that listened to my presentations I sent a personal thank you note. I maintain that practice today.

MY SPECIAL PARTNER

How could we go about identifying my alter-ego, i.e., someone with the leadership and administrative capabilities to move us to the next level? Once again, I turned to my entrepreneurial husband, and asked for his guidance. He talked with a community leader who knew of an enthusiastic and talented woman who was just completing a short term commitment with another non-profit. Randy arranged a meeting. She obliged, thinking he wanted her to identify candidates for this position. Randy, an experienced recruiter, knew that he wanted her to consider the job of partnering with his wife.

LOCAL BUSINESS PEOPLE

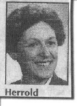

Jan Herrold has been named interim executive director of the CentralPennsylvania Health Education Center. She will continue to expand the areas of financial development, community support and public relations. Previously she was director of financial development for the YWCA. The HEC's projected opening date is September 1994.

Herrold

9-8-91

Jan Herrold came to our home and I immediately agreed with Randy's judgment. She possessed an upbeat, can-do attitude along with a tremendous history of successful leadership roles in the community. We had a very productive dialogue, in spite of the dust and dirt of a home remodeling project, and she agreed to become our Part-Time, Interim Executive Director. Her 'part-time' position instantly became a full-time obsession and it lasted three wonderful years.

Jan quickly became my colleague and co-worker, sister-in-crime and mentor. Once again, Randy knew what I needed and found a special angel. Jan possessed tremendous financial skills, could write with the legalese of an attorney and was extremely organized. We developed a wonderfully productive working partnership. I concentrated on relationship building and she concentrated on organization building. One of her first tasks was to establish a budget.

My budgeting process was an accountant's nightmare; whatever I needed I bought, then threw the receipts in one of my discarded shoe boxes. During one of our first meetings, Jan asked for my budget and I handed the shoebox to her. Nineteen years later, I'm still teased about my former "special" way of balancing a budget. To me, balancing a budget meant holding the shoe box in both hands.

Jan wrote our first business plan. Together we created our mission and vision and received board approval for these important statements. I asked people for money, Jan wrote grants for money. What a team! Rumor circulated that business leaders would identify us walking down the street toward them and they would cross to the other side because they knew we would ask them for something. We loved it! I slept better knowing that Jan was my partner and whatever I did not think to do she would. For three years, we combined our diverse skills to build curriculum and exhibits; visited numerous sites looking for the perfect location; planned and managed the renovation of a 30,000 square foot historic car dealership; and solicited over three million dollars in gifts to create the HEC.

It was the best of times for me.

An external bond between us was that her two children were the same ages as two of mine. In fact, one Saturday in early fall, we were on opposite sides of our nine year-old sons' soccer match. During the match, our sons did not see eye to eye on a particular play and proceeded to get into a shoving match. They resolved their difference quickly just like Jan and I would when we would not agree on issues. (minus the shoving)

Locating a home for "my baby" was extremely frustrating. Jan and I traveled from one end of York County to the other and beyond. During our two year and twenty-two site quest we even looked at regional possibilities in Hershey and New Cumberland, PA.

1992 - One day a community leader asked me to look at a car dealership in the south end of the city. I drove from his office to the address on South George Street. What I witnessed was a dirty, 90

year- old building with collapsed ceilings that desperately needed the mercy of a wrecking ball. I called him the next day and explained that this dilapidated building was not part of my dream. He said I was at the wrong building. I had looked at the soon-to-be razed building next door to his recommended site. I drove downtown

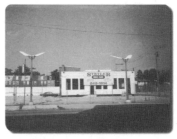
The wrong building

again to the correct site at 515 South George Street, a former auto dealership.

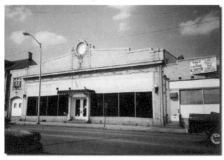
515 South George Street

As I peeked through the huge showroom windows and saw the beautiful black and white tiled floor, the oak wainscoting, and the spiral "titanic" staircase, my heart began to race. I knew that I had found "home" for the health education center. But behind the splendor of the showroom was the mechanic's area with two underground oil storage tanks and contaminated soil that had to be professionally tested and removed.

Pools of slick oil had to be side-stepped on the concrete floor as well as paint cans that lined the outside of the metal body shop where the cars and trucks had been spray-painted.

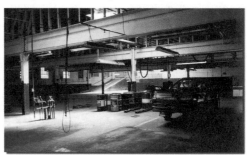
Interior of 515 South George Street

As fate would have it, at the same time, a local business owner approached Jan and myself and said that he would donate several acres of land on the north side of York near a major highway, on which we could build the HEC. (This was important because we were going to be a regional facility with students arriving from a 50 mile radius).

Now the Board had to make a very important decision; accept the free, pristine farm land north of the city or renovate a 70 year-old abandoned city building possibly containing underground toxic-filled tanks. You might think that it should have been an easy decision. In fact, it was the first hotly contested issue among our board members. Many board members wanted to accept the free land: "You never know what's behind the closed doors of a renovation project, they warned."

But Jan and I had our hearts set on 515 South George Street. We handled it like the business women we were becoming. We created a decision matrix, sent it to the Board and set a meeting date. The points in favor of the renovation were strong. The donated land needed thousands of dollars of excavation preparation. In addition, many business leaders in York wanted to continue the rejuvenation of the downtown area. They suggested that they would be inclined to be more generous during the capital campaign if we chose downtown. Jan and I loved the idea of restoring a beautiful building and wanted to be part of the revitalization efforts in the Southeast part of the city.

Because so many board members wanted to come to the meeting it was held at the public library. The Board sided with us and unanimously voted for the downtown site. I was thrilled! I finally had a building that matched the vision in my head… for a premiere, regional health education center.

GETTING THE WORD OUT

One cold, Sunday on January, 17, 1993 we threw a big party at 515 South George Street so neighboring residents and the community-at-large could see the Before and plans for the After. Volunteers were dressed as celery, strawberries, and broccoli. Yours truly was

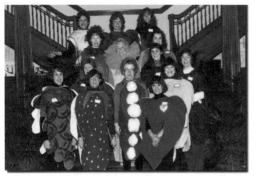

Volunteer "fruits & vegetables"

dressed in a bright red heart-shaped costume from my neck to below my knees. My real heart was pumping wildly with excitement and joy.

The Health Education Center had a home; one that needed a lot of remodeling but nonetheless a home! What a thrill to be announcing on TV and radio to my community that soon they would be welcomed and inspired in our state-of-the-art teaching theaters. What a fantastic day.

Yes, we had a home but now we needed to renovate it (one million dollars), create and pay for exhibits (one million dollars) and secure money to operate, (one million dollars). (For some reason it always seems to take a million dollars for anything.)

Even with a dedicated part-time Executive Director, a dynamic volunteer board, and my optimism, the tasks were overwhelming.

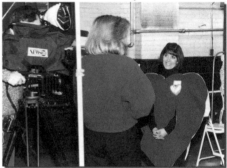

My first TV appearance

January and February days in Central Pennsylvania seem long, dark and cold. These adjectives could also describe my mood. What

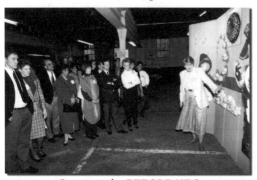

Guests at the BEFORE HEC

a let down after the glowing celebration of securing a home. Reality set in. Meeting after meeting…educational curriculum, exhibit design and creation, fundraising, fundraising, fundraising.

In the days and weeks following the site selection we traveled near and far to attend meetings upon meetings dealing with the creation of our exhibits and curriculum. Most health education centers had four teaching theaters; Family Living/Life Begins, General Health, Substance Use/Abuse and Nutrition/Fitness. But we only had money for two. So we planned to open with two teaching theaters: General Health and Family Living/Life Begins.

Very early in my process of building the board, I selected people with expertise that would assist me with the creation of exhibits and curriculum. Two committees were established: Education and Exhibit. Jan and I were joined by teachers, parents, my doctor and dentist on the Education Committee and several engineers on the Exhibit Committee. For two years we met to discuss what we were going to teach and how we would design and build our exhibits. Eventually, Jan hired a teacher from a local high school to assist with the writing of curriculum.

Members of the two committees traveled to several existing health education centers concentrating on the curriculum and exhibits; making notes on the ones that we felt were most effective teaching and demonstrating the complexities of the body.

My research of other health education centers showed that they built their exhibits and then wrote their curriculum. I wanted to do it the other way- decide what health issues were important to our community, write curriculum and then build our exhibits. We went to work gathering health statistics about York County, the State of Pennsylvania and the U. S. guidelines for school health curriculum.

As a nurse, I wanted to stress the anatomy and physiology of our bodies so people could first appreciate the miracle of their lives and then be motivated to make healthy decisions to keep their bodies working well. Jan and I were not always in harmony.

I recall one incident in which there was a significant difference of opinion. It was during one of our marathon meetings (10 hours) with our exhibit designer. I wanted two brain models for our teaching theaters: one in General Health and one in the future Substance Use/Abuse. The extra brain meant an additional $50,000.

Seven Year Pregnancy

Jan said no. We were already over budget for our exhibits. As a nurse, I felt that it was important to dramatize how alcohol depresses every part of the brain and nervous system. After all, preventing the abuse of alcohol is what got me started in the first place. I insisted and promised to find the extra money.

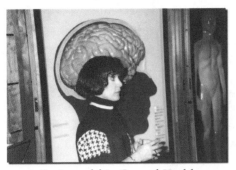

Brain model in General Health

One of our regional board members, Linda Miller, was a nurse whose husband, Bob, was the General Manager of Harley-Davidson, Inc.'s manufacturing facility, a major employer in our community. I invited them to the future home of the health education center.

As I explained to Linda and Bob about the future Substance Use/Abuse Teaching Theater I told them about the loss of my mother-in-law. I passionately expressed my desire for a huge, lighted brain exhibit. Bob was impressed with our plans. He and Linda loved the idea of teaching about the harmful effects of substances on the body's systems. They encouraged us to write a grant to Harley. Jan and I quickly submitted a grant for $250,000. It was approved and Bob Miller took great delight in riding his roaring Harley into our building to deliver the first of five $50,000 checks. What an enormous gift! The brain and the entire Substance Abuse Teaching Theater, that I had set my heart on, would happen. I didn't know that angels road motorcycles.

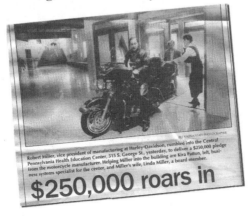

Robert Miller, vice president of manufacturing at Harley-Davidson, rumbled into the Central Pennsylvania Health Education Center, 515 S. George St., yesterday, to deliver a $250,000 pledge from the motorcycle manufacturer. Helping Miller into the building are Kira Patton, left, business systems specialist for the center, and Miller's wife, Linda Miller, a board member.

$250,000 roars in

Health can be a controversial subject especially in the sensitive area of human sexuality. Many board and committee discussions were held to determine how far the Byrnes Health Education Center would go with the delicate subject of contraception. Several ob-gyn physicians believed that this instruction should be included in our curriculum. But other members of the education committee thought that it should not be included. The Board adopted a policy that stated our curriculum would be abstinence based because this best represented the conservative mores of our community.

We continued writing curriculum for our exhibits that were being built in West Nyack, NY. This entailed many long trips to view our not-so-completed exhibits. I need to explain. Up until now, all health education centers in the country used Richard Rush Studios to build their exhibits.

We were the first health education center to send a RFP (a request for proposal) to exhibit makers. We interviewed each of them in York prior to awarding our contract. Mr. Rush was surprised that he did not get the job. I give a lot of credit to our Exhibit Committee for widening the net for exhibit creators...but the process of getting our exhibits built was considerably lengthened because the new exhibit makers were not as experienced. Still, I wouldn't have done it any other way; we wanted our health education curriculum and exhibits to be unique and to reflect the health needs of our community.

Days and weeks became months and months. This growing health education center was taking a huge amount of my time and energy.

As with most pregnancies, one can feel the pressure of the growing fetus as you carry an extra fifteen pounds that presses on and displaces internal organs. That growth process can lead to feeling uncomfortable as well as to indigestion and gas pains. I too felt the pressure of carrying the "extra" weight of the health education center in my heart and soul.

On the days when my "indigestion" would flare-up, I would do what an early advocate had advised: "… be like Woody Hayes, the Ohio State football coach,' put your head down and go for ten yards, not a touchdown.'" Some days I wanted to keep my head under my pillow, forget going for one yard.

When I experienced these difficult days, I reflected on the words of wisdom that Randy had said to me in the waning days of my third pregnancy; "this is your last opportunity to help God with a miracle."

RAISING THE MONEY

In the spring of 1992, the Board hired a professional fund-raising company to conduct a capital campaign feasibility study to identify if there was community support to raise three million dollars. This study was recommended by the Capital Campaign Review Committee of York; a group of business leaders who guide the process of large community solicitations. The committee generously supports and usually leads these county-wide fund-raisers.

When the health education center had its turn "at court" we presented our case on paper and with props. I wanted to demonstrate the effective teaching methods of using hands-on exhibits and learning by doing. So I demonstrated a show-and-tell with a REAL heart. Then I asked several members to listen to their hearts with my purple stethoscope. (I don't know if my presentation was before or after lunch.)

Committee members are still talking about seeing a real heart even today. The heart exhibit worked its magic and we were approved for a capital campaign. But the bad news was that we had to spend $8,000 of our seed money to be informed by a professional fund raising organization that we would raise less than one million dollars, based on their survey of business leaders.

I was devastated. This amount of money would not even pay for renovations. I also surmised that the professional fund-raisers received a substantial amount of money for their expertise to "guide" us. We clearly were going to do all the work of securing the financial gifts and pledges. That scenario was untenable.

Randy, Jan and I spent an entire rainy Saturday making our plans to conduct our own capital campaign for $1.75M. We worked those grueling plans for the next ten months. The fund-raising company lost a customer. An army of community volunteers persuaded, coerced and begged its way to gather large and small gifts to establish the Health Education Center. Day after day, week after week.

We had campaign chairs from the business, dental and medical professions along with the general community. Doctors asked doctors for pledges, business leaders asked business leaders. Jan wrote grants. I asked everyone for money... I even picked the pockets of family members. (Fundraising hint: never be too proud to beg from anyone.)

In September of 1993, Randy and I held a combined 20th wedding anniversary party and an end of campaign party at our home. Hundreds of people worked tirelessly for a year to gather gifts so my dream would become a reality. On our back porch, to a thrilling drum roll, campaign leaders held numbers high over their heads. $2,023,382 was pledged! We had done it! Dreams do come true. I remember the joy in my heart as members of the York community and my family dined and danced under the stars.

What a mystical, magical evening!

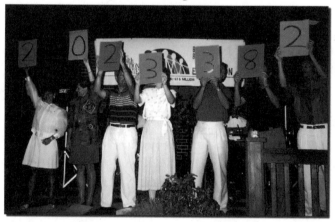

Campaign leaders demonstrating our success

But, the glow of success was short-lived. Our financial committee, led by Jim Bergdoll, soon realized that the capital campaign pledges were spread over five years and we had to pay for renovations and exhibits in year one. To bridge this financial gap, we went back to the community with a plan for creating bonds to finance us. Again the generosity of York manifested itself as we raised $750,000. We utilized municipal bonds that were callable in seven years and payable in ten. (Aren't you impressed with this nurse's financial knowledge?) The good news was we could pay our bills; the bad, we were in debt for $750,000 and every year we had to pay six (6%) percent interest to our eighteen bondholders. (this was the first time a not-for-profit had ever done this type of creative financing)

This was going to be a huge strain on our operating budget. An unspoken concern between Jan and me was the fact that we really did not know for sure if the school superintendents were actually going to authorize the funds for their students to attend our teaching facility. Where were we going to get an additional $45,000 every year to pay the interest to our bond holders? More sleepless nights.

CONSTRUCTION BEGINS

On a bright and beautiful April morning, 1994, Jan and I were assisted by twenty 5-yr-old children as we broke ground for the renovations to the former car dealership at 515 South George Street. Actually, we had a huge sledge hammer and we smacked it into the side of the building that we were razing. What fun.

The construction process was never ending: interviewing architects, hiring an architect, reviewing blueprints, arguing with the architect, selecting a contractor, reviewing the bid, arguing with the con-tractor. I experienced worry, fear, doubt and frustration but never regret that I had

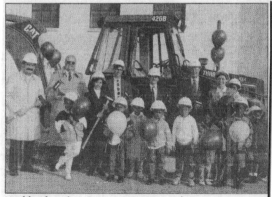

Health Education Center starts renovations

The Central PA Health Education Center celebrated the start of renovations to the former D.E. Stetler and Sons building in York with children from the Crispus Attucks Day Care Center taking part in the celebration. Shown with the children are, from left to right, James K. Bergdoll, vice president, board of directors; Mayor Charles Robertson; Susan P. Byrnes, R.N., president, board of directors; Frank Dittenhafer, architect; Daren Sealover, C.M., Kinsley Construction; Sen. Michael E. Bortner; and Jan Herrold, executive director. The center is scheduled to open early in 1995, offering programs to school-aged children that will supplement and enhance classroom instruction.

started down the path of building a health education center.

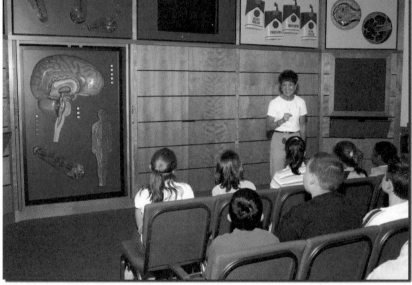

An enthusiastic educator in one of dramatic teaching theaters

One reason I did not have regret is that my dreams kept me going. I could envision our teaching theaters filled with excited children learning about their bodies using larger than life models of hearts, brains, lungs and teeth. They would be having fun while they discovered the wonders of life. These students would take their health education home to their parents and together they would become inspired to make healthy choices for the rest of their lives.

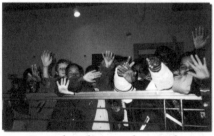

Excited students ready to make healthy choices

But there were those who wanted to crush my dream…

One high school Superintendent I met with sat back in his big leather chair, put his hands together and said, "So what do you get out of this? Will you create a place where you can have a job?" I tried to keep my Italian temper in check and coolly responded that I was volunteering my time and that I would continue to do so until my dream became a reality. The same Superintendent was quoted in our local newspaper as saying, "How good can this educational idea be if an educator did not think of it?" Unfortunately, this superintendent is still working in education, albeit, at a university.

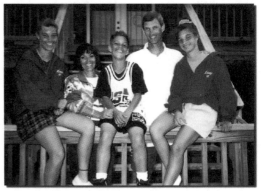

Byrnes family at the Outer Banks,
North Carolina

We were now into year four of the pregnancy. My children were 13, 12, and 11.

DISASTROUS DIRECTOR DECISION

Even with all this excitement and progress, Jan and I were growing weary. Jan's part-time interim position had begun in June 1991. She had worked full-time for a part-time salary for three years (what a magnificent personal gift). The lion's share of the work was completed, or so we thought. Jan announced that she would be leaving and that we should search for a new Director who could take the HEC forward.

After a laborious search process, the Board hired a state employed health educator in July, 1994. It took me only five days to know that we had made a grave mistake. The new Executive Director took tons of renovation pictures but little was getting accomplished. I began 'management triage' by assigning specific tasks to be accomplished on a timeline.

Deadlines came and went. I shared my concerns with Randy and members of our Executive Committee. Some accused me of not being able to give up my "baby". Others dismissed my comments and suggested that it could be a personality conflict. Both perceptions were inaccurate.

We were at a critical phase of our development and I was not going to jeopardize the work of so many people. We consulted with an attorney who reviewed all of my documentation.

With the attorney's guidance, we asked for the Executive Director's resignation five weeks after he began. He reluctantly agreed. To my dismay, it was suggested that we give him severance pay to ensure that there would not be any unpleasant backlash. This money had to come from the gifts that we had gathered to build the HEC. It was a very low emotional time for me.

The Board voted that I should become the Interim Executive Director. This was a very busy and important time in our development. People had to be hired to teach our health education programs and the renovations and exhibits needed to be completed. The Board and Advisory Board were very supportive and Jan graciously stayed by my side for several more months but the BUCK STOPPED WITH ME.

MORE MOTHER'S GUILT

At the same time, I attempted to maintain my role as a responsible mother. One summer day, my two jobs clashed. I was told that my daughter Katie was on line 2. I said "Hi", but immediately sensed trouble. She told me that her brother had been thrown from his dirt bike. A neighbor was driving him to me. As I said good-bye, I could see the car pull up in front of our building. I rushed to the car where Dan was sitting in the front seat holding his right arm close to his ribs. I instantly recognized the fractured right clavicle protruding from the skin. Carefully, we transferred him to my car. I drove quickly and carefully to the Emergency Department, my former place of employment. An X-ray confirmed the break. As Dan lay on the stretcher waiting to be fitted with a sling, he dozed from the pain medicine. My eyes filled with tears; my heart heavy with guilt. Would this have happened if I had been home instead of at another endless meeting?

Was the Health Education Center really so important? I was volunteering hours upon hours of time away from my children to help other children.

That night as I lay in Randy's arms, I shared my guilt and tears. How could I continue to take so much time and energy away from our family? Randy reassured me that our three children were doing just fine. Someday, they would be very proud of their mother and the Health Education Center. I had my doubts.

It was September 1994.

The non-paying job responsibilities of being Chair of the Board and Executive Director were time consuming and overwhelming. I was juggling HEC obligations and the hectic schedules of three teenagers. My life was unbalanced. I could not even the find time to go to the grocery store.

Reality was, I did not have the time or energy to be an understanding wife or mother, much less, time for extended family or friends. The irony of it was, I wasn't making personal healthy choices. I was a wreck.

MOVING DAY

In November of '94 the Central PA Health Education Center was scheduled to move from Randy's office to our renovated 515 South George Street. The move was planned for the Friday after Thanksgiving. On moving day Jan was on a well deserved vacation with her family. Our senior employee was unhappy with an internal situation and only came to help for one hour. So the job fell to me, a second employee and a group of temporary workers. As we maneuvered furniture in the pouring rain I called Randy and asked him to please come and help me because some of the temp workers were more interested in trying to impress me with long stories rather than move desks.

As we began to unload at our new home, it was evident much work still needed to be completed: saw horses and piles of dust in the Great Hall, tools and equipment everywhere and an eight-page construction punch list.

At around 3:00 P.M., I stood alone in the shell of my dream: partially painted walls, missing exhibits, unfinished teaching theaters, a skeleton staff with no Executive Director and a $750,00 debt. I was overwhelmed with fatigue and fear. I had been leaving my family and volunteering full-time for five years.

How could this possibly succeed? It was one of the lowest points in my crusade to establish a health education center.

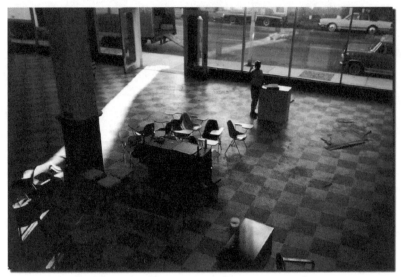

Great HalL, 515 S. George St., on moving day

The Christmas of 1994 came and went. Normally, we do it all: decorate two live trees; make gingerbread houses and cookies with the kids and their friends and bake banana nut bread for family and neighbors. I love Christmas and usually enjoy the holiday spirit for weeks. But this year I was numb. I lay on the couch as Randy and our three teenagers trimmed one little tree in our family room.

I did not have the energy to celebrate Christmas with my family. What had I done?

4

Birth: We came alive in '95

The physical exhaustion that pervades a nine month pregnancy is quickly forgotten in the serenity of the moment when the new mother cuddles the tiny gift from God.

In late January, 1995, I felt this warm after-glow, when we launched eight pilot programs in our General Health and Family Living Teaching Theaters. Hundreds of children were streaming through our bright red doors to learn about their magnificent bodies and how and why to keep them WELL. Our educators produced magical health education with the lighted brain that was taller than many of our students and the heart/lung fiber optic model that visualized de-oxygenated blood from the heart atriums traveling to the lungs, picking up oxygen, returning to the heart ventricles and then pumping the blood to the rest of the body.

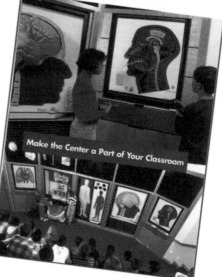

Students and teachers alike were oooing and aaahing as they learned by seeing, hearing and doing. We were making a difference and it was wonderful.

After seven years, with hundreds of experts holding my hand during the conception, development and painful 'labor and delivery' phases, my baby was born. To describe my state of mind as euphoric was putting it mildly.

The dust was settling in our regional teaching facility

General Health Teaching Theater

but the eight-page construction punch list (unfinished details) needed to be addressed. Fortunately, a very special and knowledgeable board member, Jack Deroche, took this grueling task from my extensive to-do list. He took charge of all meetings with our construction manager and supervised the tedious work of finishing every incomplete construction task. This angel, was wearing a tool belt! To this day, I loathe renovation projects.

During the past hectic months, my untested managerial skills had produced more than one anxious moment both for me and our new employees. One day, one of our three teachers accompanied me for a short drive to our local bank branch. I was making a deposit for payroll. She looked at me, as we turned into the parking area, and gently queried "You really don't have much experience being an Executive Director, do you?" She was a nurse also and had borne witness to my inexperience with many of the managerial tasks of a fledgling non-profit. As Chair of the Board and Executive Director, I was responsible for: payroll and accounting, creating the personnel manual, addressing the needs of the staff, leading committee and board meetings, developing strategy for our annual giving campaign...even finding someone to clean our building. Because of my German mother's lessons from home I was organized and efficient but I lacked the know-how of business management. In my world, if you saw something that needed to be done, you did it. This initiative is fine in start-up mode but can become a source of chaos in an expanding organization. I thought I was doing ok. I didn't realize that my incompetence was transparent and affecting the staff negatively.

It was March, 1995. Five months into my dual role of Interim Executive Director and Chair of the Board, my health was suffering ... mentally and physically. I felt that I was not being an effective Board Chair, Executive Director, wife or mother. Randy said that it was time to get away. Sanibel Island, FL. was the destination for our family for a week of rest & relaxation. I remember my teenagers wrestling with one another on the sofa. The sound of their laughter rejuvenated my spirits. The girls were in training for spring soccer so they ran every day with their soccer coach/dad. Dan would join them in a fun family game of soccer in the sand and I would breathe in the nourishment of their voices at play. I relaxed in a beach chair and could literally feel my strength return. Seeing and hearing the waves crash on the surf created a sense of peacefulness in me. I could feel my mind, body and spirit becoming calm and returning to balance.

Back at 515 South George Street, I was missing my first board meeting in seven years.

Looking back, perhaps Jan had called Randy and asked him to get me out of town. The Board passed a unanimous resolution to change the name of the Central PA Health Education Center to the Susan P. Byrnes Health Education Center.

When I returned to my office, a beautiful spring bouquet adorned my desk. (I love flowers.) In my hasty style of reading, I read the card which said "from the Board in appreciation for seven years of volunteer leadership and dedication to the **Susan P. Byrnes Health Education Center**. The new name didn't register. When I called Jan to thank her she asked me if I had read the card. Yes, I said. She patiently asked me to reread it. I slowly read the card. Oh my, what an honor and privilege! It moved me to tears. Because of the efforts of hundreds of people, I would be leaving a legacy for my beloved community. What a dream come true!

Shortly after our next board meeting it was suggested that I begin a search for Executive Director # 4. (I was #3)

I remember responding that I was too busy to undertake this process alone so a search committee was formed. We received many resumes in response to our ads. We made telephone calls and conducted initial exploratory interviews. Following our earlier debacle with #2 (our five-week Executive Director), I was more than slightly anxious about this process.

Sam Bressi, a young, energetic and entrepreneurial manager from Hershey Medical Center agreed to be our Executive Director after much pleading from yours truly. I need to explain why I was groveling like Miss Hoolihan in "Annie." Keep in mind as you read my explanation that I am a nurse, not an HR Director. But come to think of it, I don't know why I was the contact person. I should have left it to Bill, the HR Director of a large corporation who was on our committee and the expert on these matters. Why didn't we think of that, Bill?

The search committee was basically at an impasse on the two finalists. One was a female R.N. who had worked her way into a leadership position at a local hospital, the other was Sam, with an MBA, and five years experience as manager of the Hershey Medical Fitness Center.

We decided to offer the position to the female R.N. Here is where I made a grave mistake. I called Sam first and told him that he was sooo close to being our first choice but an offer would be extended to the other candidate. He wasn't happy but he was professional in his understanding. Then, I called the R.N. who proceeded to say that she didn't think that she was the right person to lead the Health Education Center.

OOPS!

I called Sam back immediately and began to sing his praises and begged him to consider becoming our Executive Director. Did you notice that his name ended in a vowel? His Italian temper and bruised ego flared. I coaxed and cajoled like my life depended on it. He finally agreed to bring his wife and two small children to the Center that coming Sunday afternoon. (I hoped that I could charm his wife and children)

During his family's visit I sensed that Sam and his wife Linda were fascinated with our two dramatic teaching theaters and the HEC's potential impact on the health of children and their families in our region. When Sam had been interviewed, he had outlined a visionary five-year plan for the HEC. During this Sunday visit he again talked about his plan. It became clearer to me that Sam was the entrepreneur that we needed to take this nascent organization to new heights. Linda and I hit it off immediately. Had this visit convinced Sam to believe in my dream and take it beyond my expectations? Was he willing to leave the security of an established medical center and move his young family to York to lead a fledgling not-for-profit? Sam decided to think about it for awhile.

It was April, 1995…

…time to dedicate the Susan P. Byrnes Health Education Center and honor all of the people who helped to make it a reality.

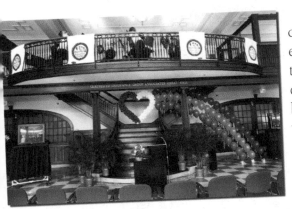

Our Beautiful Glatfelter Great Hall

What an awesome celebration! Friday evening was a private thank you for the hundreds of dedicated board members and volunteers who had devoted their time, talents and treasures to build a special place for the community to learn about staying healthy. Our beautiful Glatfelter Great Hall sparkled with sun streaming through the antique, leaded glass windows. The heavenly scent of huge bouquets of flowers; many containing white roses (York is the White Rose City), sent by well-wishers wafted in the air.

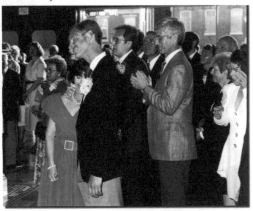

Tears of joy

The chimes of clinking glasses by volunteers congratulating each other and music from a high school orchestra created a fairy-tale atmosphere. A high school friend sang "Climb Every Mountain" at my request (I had been singing this to myself for seven years). There wasn't a dry eye in the joyous crowd.

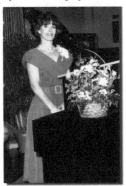

My thank you speech

In my short welcome and thank you address, I shared the story of Pollyanna, one of my favorite movies. Pollyanna was a young girl who came to a small town to live after her missionary parents died. She stayed with a very strict Aunt Polly who could not suppress Pollyanna's joy of life. This young girl spread her happiness to the entire community. The evening of the Fourth of July celebration,

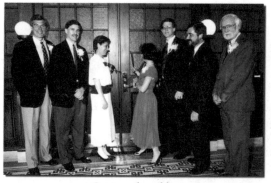

Cutting the ribbon

(Aunt Polly forbade her niece to attend) Pollyanna fell as she was sneaking out of her second floor bedroom. She broke her back. The day she was leaving to go to a big town for surgery everyone came to Aunt Polly's home to wish Pollyanna well. I felt like Pollyanna, the whole town had come to our Great Hall to celebrate my dream come true!

The next morning, a Saturday, under beautiful sunny skies we cut the ribbon for our first Annual Family Health Festival. Hundreds of children, parents and grandparents filled our teaching theaters, the Great Hall and spilled out into our parking lot. What a festive day. Together, families had fun while they learned how and why they needed to take

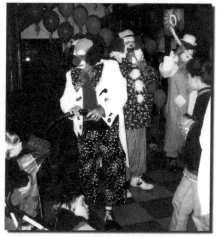

First Family Health Festival

special care of their bodies. They were inspired to make healthy choices. My heart and soul were glowing.

My HEC baby was christened!

My own babies had also grown up: Katie 17, Kristy 15, and Dan 14. (Do you remember how old they were in the beginning of this story?)

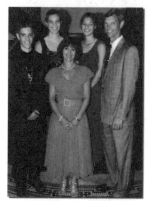

April, 1995
The Byrnes Family

Birth: We came alive in '95

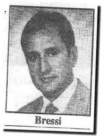

Bressi

June 1, 1995, Sam and Linda Bressi took a leap of faith. Sam accepted the job and the Bressi angels moved to York and Sam became the fourth Executive Director of the Susan P. Byrnes Health Education Center. (Byrnes HEC) In reality, he is #1, our first full-time, salaried executive. (Sam will love that I refer to him as #1) After his first month of working, Sam jokingly shared with me that he was concerned that he might be asked to resign during his fifth week of employment... do you remember what happened to our #2 Executive Director?

Like most newborn's, including my own, the Byrnes HEC went through times of colic, sleepless nights, and inevitable crying. Poor Sam never had the opportunity to enjoy a honeymoon with his new position; the need for leadership immediately surfaced.

A negative administrative assistant immediately began to go behind Sam's back and tell me that he was doing a poor job with our finances; that he always needed to whip out his little calculator to do math and therefore he must not be very smart. I laughed this off. Sam does have an MBA. He didn't understand our finances? Who could possibly understand our deficit budget? We had little income and large expenditures including a $750,000 bond debt that required annual interest payments of $45,000. Sam could read the writing on the wall and he was nervous.

I tried to reassure Sam that I was going to raise the money so we could balance this precarious budget. He seemed very skeptical especially when I forgot to complete the paperwork to establish his new medical insurance package with us thereby leaving him and his family with no medical coverage. After this managerial fumbling, Sam later told me that he had confided with Linda that he had made a serious mistake leaving the security of a large hospital to come to a small non-profit.

And it wasn't just our serious money shortage...

A major staff debacle occurred six months after Sam started. During their monthly meeting the woman who showed signs of disrespect to Sam said that he was doing a terrible job as Executive Director and the three other staff members agreed. MUTINY!

Sam was furious. That afternoon it began to snow. The bad weather lasted for forty-eight hours.

Everyone was snowed-in for three days. I'll never forget the myriad of highly charged phone calls between Sam and me. As Board Chair I emphatically supported him. But as a new boss he was reluctant to fire them. For nine months as Executive Director I had dealt with these three employees and their negativity, lack of cooperation, and disrespect. Only the fourth was truly upbeat and enjoyed her work. How dare they try to take over and undermine Sam. My temper got the best of me and I offered these heated words of advice to Sam, "Meet with them individually and tell them to either put their oar in your boat or get the hell out." That is exactly what he did. One was fired, one resigned and one moved out of town. It was now up to Sam to create his own team.

This mutiny was my fault. I should have handled these unpleasant personnel issues prior to Sam's start. (Hind-sight is always 20/20; unless you are over fifty and then it might require visual assistance.) However, if I had fired the staff I would have become the de facto Executive Director, education staff, Business Coordinator and Board Chair. That would have pushed me over the edge. I failed miserably as manager of the Byrnes HEC and Sam inherited a mess.

The wonder of it all is that Sam and I worked magically together. Sam concentrated on recruiting staff and getting students in our teaching theaters. I threw all my energy into creating a tremendous board and gathering thousands and thousands of dollars to balance our budget. At times, we joked with one another that our working relationship was much like a marriage. In truth, some weeks we spent more time together than we did with our respective spouses and family. With Sam as the paid Executive Director I NOW KNEW, the buck stopped with him. I was the volunteer... Sam was being paid the big bucks (or as big as we could afford) to endure the sleepless nights.

One of the Byrnes HEC's very special moments occurred in October, 1995, when Dr. C. Everett Koop, M.D., the former Surgeon General of the United States from 1980-1989 visited our facility. At the time, he was the Honorary Chair of the national SAFE KIDS Initiative and was in town as the guest of York Hospital, to

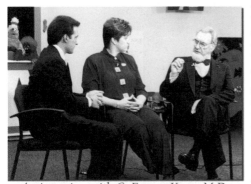

An interview with C. Everett Koop, M.D.

kick-off a local SAFE KIDS effort. Upon learning that he would be visiting our community, Sam and I set about trying to arrange for him to witness our brand new teaching facility. Much to our delight he and his wife agreed to tour the Byrnes HEC following his luncheon address. Imagine our mix of pride and trepidation when one of the most distinguished physicians in the country walked through our double red doors. This was the building that three short years ago had been housing the remnants of an auto body paint shop and was now filled with children learning about the wonders of the human body. As we tiptoed into the Family Living/Life Begins Teaching Theater our vivacious Health Educator was explaining to a class of fifth grade students the concept of twins. One of the children asked about Siamese twins. Dr. Koop, corrected the child, stepped to the front of the class of fifty students and described how as a pediatric surgeon he had actually separated co-joined twins at Children's Hospital of Philadelphia. You could almost feel the excitement pulsing through the veins of the staff, Sam and the little nurse from Spry. My mind flashed to so many memories of returning to my silent home after late night presentations and my children already asleep, innumerable meetings, challenges that had seemed insurmountable and now I'm watching the former Surgeon General of the United States patiently and with great care explain the miracle of life to a class of children in York, PA.

If I was breathing, I didn't know it.

Following Dr. Koop's impromptu teaching moment we moved to our General Health Teaching Theater. As he reviewed our models and listened to our curriculum content he exclaimed, "You have finally found a way to put pizzazz into prevention!" In that moment Sam and a beaming five-foot nurse turned tour guide, were filled with a joy and pride that was palpable. Dr. Koop is the Father of Prevention and the Byrnes Health Education Center had just received the Koop Seal of Approval.

I started breathing again!

5

Striving for Excellence

EXCELLENCE can be attained if you
CARE more than others think is WISE...
RISK more that others think is SAFE...
DREAM more than others think is PRACTICAL...
EXPECT more that others think is POSSIBLE.
— Anonymous

The next phase of the Byrnes HEC, and its leadership, was not as much about survival as success. Sam Bressi had proven to be an excellent choice as our President/CEO. As the Board of Directors, especially our Executive Committee, and Sam, developed in their roles we began to witness the fruits of our efforts. Sam maximized his talents through both his leadership skills and the selection of a tremendously enthusiastic and competent staff. The Board supported his efforts and the presence of the Byrnes HEC became a fixture in our community.

For seven years, Sam and I worked side-by-side to build the premiere regional resource for quality health education programs. We demanded excellence of ourselves, board and staff. More and more schools brought their students to experience our dynamic teachers and programs. In only our second year of operation, we balanced our budget. This was accomplished through the combination of program fees and the generosity of our community supporting our annual HeartBeat Scholarship Program. Businesses not only contributed money but began to contract with our Wellness Works Programs for their employees.

From the moment I decided to pursue my dream for a health education center, I wanted to teach children AND adults.

The Wellness Works Committee started meeting immediately after we opened our first two teaching theaters in 1995. For six years we planned, conducted marketing surveys with local businesses and adjusted to several false starts. The Board believed in my thinking that to truly affect behavioral change you must educate parents and children simultaneously. Board members voted to continue to financially support corporate/adult programs in spite of many lean years. In 2006, for the first time, Wellness Works

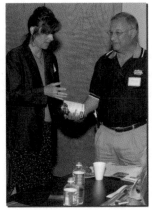

Wellness Works

produced above budget. The demand for adult programs keeps growing. I am convinced that when families are educated about the importance of how their bodies work and how they can keep them working well, they are more likely to act on this knowledge; to buy green vegetables instead of processed foods at the grocery store, to turn off the TV and go play outside or to refuse to smoke. The Byrnes HEC is one of a handful of health education centers in the country that has health education programs for children and adults...the FULL CIRCLE.

PARTNERSHIPS are the core of our success:

Bressi and Byrnes
Board and Staff
Byrnes HEC and businesses/individuals
Byrnes HEC and other not-for-profits

We were living the thrills and challenges of our infant and toddler years.

The following were some of the highlights:

1995   We open our bright red doors
       Former US Surgeon General C. Everett Koop visits
       Annual HeartBeat Scholarship established

1996   Harley-Davidson, Inc. funds SubstanceUse/ Abuse Theater.

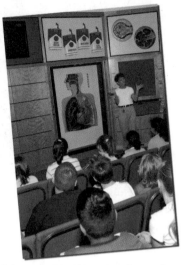

Substance Use/AbuseTeaching Theater

The Byrnes HEC welcomes its 50,000th participant

1997   Rotary District 7390 adopts the Byrnes HEC as a District
Project providing financial support and volunteers

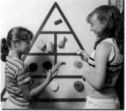

1998 Nutrition and Fitness, our fifth
Teaching Theater opens
Byrnes HEC establishes Corporate
Wellness Works Programs

*Nutrition and Fitness
Theater*

The Byrnes HEC welcomes its 100,000th participant

1999   Byrnes HEC creates Discovery Carts, hands-on activities to
reinforce and extend what children learn in the teaching
theaters.

2000   Penn State University evaluates our programs
Summer Camps begin
Planned Giving Committee establishes endowment fund

Birth: We came alive in '95

The Byrnes HEC welcomes its 150,000th participant

2001   Mildred Gabrielson Body Shop for Early Learners re-opens
Simon, a seven foot tall, deep purple muppet becomes our mascot

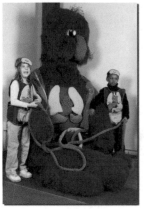

Simon and friends

2002   Learning Labs, outreach teaching begins

The Byrnes HEC welcomes its 300,000th participant

2003   *e*-Learning initiative develops five health education lesson plans.

2004   BYRNES HEC REPAYS ITS BOND DEBT, (WOW, WE ARE DEBT FREE!)

2005   Circle of Heart Endowment grows to 80 members

May 26th, the Byrnes HEC welcomes its 500,000th participant

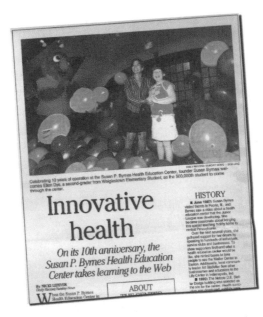

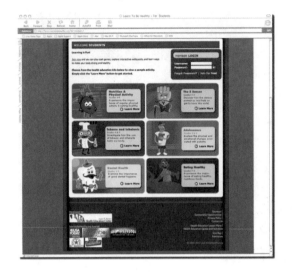

2006 **www.LearntobeHealthy.org**

In January, 2006, the Byrnes HEC officially launches its
e-Learning website LearntobeHealthy.org.
LearntobeHealthy.org represents the culmination of years
of effort to develop a high-quality, innovative educational
tool enabling the Center to reach far beyond the region
with the message of healthy living. In only a few short
months it had won two prestigious awards for innovation.

The Center welcomes its 600,000th Participant

National Impact

By the end of 2006, LearntobeHealthy.org's membership tops
12,000 with users from every state in the Nation and 168 countries
around the globe. The educational website has now been recognized by several national organizations including USA Today and
Highlights magazine.

A significant step in the evolution of any organization is the
establishment of a succession plan for leadership. For thirteen
years, 1989-2002, I had volunteered as the Board Chair of the
Byrnes HEC. In 2002, when the HEC was seven years old, I knew

both personally and organizationally it was time to step aside. ("A good leader knows when to get out of the way of her growing organization.") Much as a parent intuitively knows when it is time for a child to establish his/her own destiny, it was time for our maturing entity to embrace a formal succession plan of Board leadership.

For eight months, Sam, our Executive Committee and I worked on a Strategic Plan that could be a template for our future. This effort culminated with a full-day strategic session involving our combined fifty-seven advisory and board members and staff. We had attained our initial Mission and Vision and been balancing the budget since year two. We had developed health education programs that were not only impacting our community but were literally available world-wide through the internet.

As we contemplated the breadth of our impact on educating and inspiring children and adults to make healthy choices, we clearly recognized there was much to be done.

We created a new Mission and Vision and completely deconstructed and rebuilt our business model. Four separate platform areas were created: Theater, Outreach, e-Learning and Planned Giving. Each business platform area was chaired by a board member. In effect, my responsibilities as Chair of the Board were divided into five leadership positions. I retained only one of them - Planned Giving.

During the wrap-up meeting, four men were introduced who had graciously agreed to accept the newly created leadership positions. I took the opportunity to thank our new leaders and everyone for being a part of this exciting but exhausting strategic process. I must have been experiencing brain drain because I heard myself saying: "it appears to me that it will take four men to do the work one woman has been doing for thirteen years.

It brought down the house with laughter and love.

The culture of the Byrnes HEC is simply a version of The Golden Rule, Treat others like you would like to be treated. And remember that no one is more important than the Mission and Vision. What do I mean? Internally, we say that we are FIERCELY INDEPENDENT. To maintain this independence we must always be

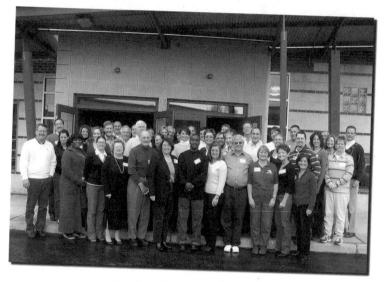

Board and staff strategic planning session

financially strong. Additionally, no one, no matter how much time or money he/she gives to the Byrnes HEC, is more important than the Mission and Vision. I have shared with Sam that even if I, the Founder, ever behaved in a manner that disrespected this culture that we had built, he should take my key away.

Because of this culture it has become almost easy to garner dedicated individuals from the community to serve on our boards and to recruit enthusiastic staff. We are the Byrnes HEC family that works hand-in-hand with the York and surrounding communities to make our world HEALTHIER and a better place to live, work and play.

"We can do no great things, only small things with great love."

Mother Teresa

6

YOU "R" Your Community

A __Community__ isn't something that you are part of; it's something that is **part of you.**

Plato

HOW GIVING CHANGED ME

As I reflect on my life, I see a pattern of responding to situations with feelings of deep passion and then going into action. Nine times out of ten this has been a good thing; I see someone in need and I help them. Usually, my heart responds before my head. Fortunately, these sometimes rash decisions didn't cause me to lose my head, just a little self-esteem. My standing operating procedures are to live the golden rule and believe in the power of one.

Leading the charge to build the Byrnes Health Education Center allowed me to put my passion for prevention into action; helping thousands of others and strengthening my conviction that one person can make a difference, with the support and commitment of her community.

In my wildest imagination, I never dreamed how joyous my life would be. During moments of reflection, especially during yoga, tears of gratitude spring spontaneously to my brown eyes.

Through the apparently dissimilar acts of giving and receiving one can reap immeasurable joy. As I reflect on my roles in the development of the Byrnes Health Education Center I am continually struck by the love and friendship that I have received from hundreds of generous givers in our special community.

As with most gifts, there is always a price to be paid. After nineteen years of building my dream, I have incurred the requisite grey hairs (carefully disguised by my stylist) and while my stature in the community may have grown, the natural aging process has reduced my frame by $1/2$ an inch. Standing tall has become a bit of an oxymoron.

In addition to these physical changes, I have experienced noticeable shifts in both my mind and spirit.

As you may recall, I'm the nurse who kept all her receipts in a shoebox in those formative years. Thankfully, through trial and error, along with impromptu financial tutoring sessions by Jim Bergdoll and Sam Bressi, I learned not only the value of a budget but how to use its contents in my solicitation meetings with financially astute philanthropists. I also came to appreciate that when wearing the hat of an Executive Director it is important to think first with the head and then the heart even though I knew my passion for prevention was ultimately "the wind beneath my wings" at many a financial meeting.

My intellect has been stretched beyond what I thought I was capable of comprehending. Experts in business, finance and education were my mentors as together we built a small organization. I began to think like an entrepreneur. Even when engaged in completely unrelated activities I found my thoughts drifting to the Health Education Center. Now I understood why it was so hard for Randy to switch gears when he came home from the office. There is something to "walking in another's shoes" to be able to see the world from his perspective. My admiration and respect for my entrepreneurial husband had grown tremendously.

As the Health Education Center began to be recognized in the community so did my leadership ability. It was never a goal of mine to become a "mover and shaker" (other than on the dance floor), it just happened. I was too busy juggling my roles as wife, mother and Chair of the Board to ponder what others were thinking about me.

In my Byrnes HEC role, I loved the interactions with people from all walks of life. It was exhilarating to learn how to conduct a business meeting, demonstrate how exhibits worked, conduct a capital campaign and have York residents say "YES", they wanted to keep each other WELL. Gathering everyone's energy, time and talents to build a place where people can learn how and why to take charge of their health continually fueled my passion for prevention. What a thrill to encourage others to truly recognize that life is a gift and it is our responsibility to take good care of it.

A few years after we opened our bright red doors, a board member came to me following a meeting and said," I finally get it." He could see that I was puzzled and he continued, with a huge smile on his face, "After all these years of listening to you talk about prevention I finally understand your enthusiasm. I stopped smoking several years ago at the behest of my son. I have lost twenty pounds and I feel great!"

(*Did you know* that for every pound of fat we add to our body it has to produce 200 miles of blood vessels to nourish this adipose tissue?)

I was ecstatic. This dear friend took charge of his health and made several healthy lifestyle changes. Imagine, loosing just 10 pounds of fat means that your heart would have a much easier time of pumping blood around your body. A change in behavior like this can extend a person's life and perhaps prevent disease even a premature death.

Not long after my conversation with this friend, my community surprised me. I was asked to be the Grand Marshall for our County's Halloween Parade. Thirty years earlier I had marched in this same event with my high school band. I was thrilled to have my parents, wearing their Byrnes Health Education Center sweat shirts, sitting below me in the bright orange, convertible lead car. This honor the community had given

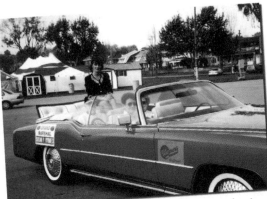

to me made me realize that I had made a difference. Like my board member the community was beginning to embrace a passion for prevention.

Bright orange lead car

As mentioned earlier, I lived by the golden rule both as a nurse and in my relationships that were created through the Byrnes HEC. Never did I anticipate that so many gentle strangers would, in a myriad of ways, impact and enhance my life's journey. I thrive on the pleasure of helping others. Performing an unexpected act of kindness, doing something nice for someone and most of all, helping individuals appreciate their gift of life is my life's work. The creation of the Byrnes Health Education Center was the ultimate in helping others, stretching my mind and allowing me to influence and impact others as a leader. My satisfaction comes when I know that someone has become inspired to truly love herself, take charge of her health and make healthy choices.

PASSION CHANGES MY COMMUNITY

Year after year, as I attended hundreds of committee and board meetings at the Byrnes Health Education Center and the South George Street Community Partnership, I began to witness a transformation of South George Street; the Byrnes Health Education Center was the first building to be renovated. Families began to move into the beautiful red brick homes, the decaying cab company building next to our parking lot was demolished and the beautiful two-story Loretta Clayborn Building was built by the Crispus Attucks Association. This building was named in honor of a local woman who has been nationally recognized for her accomplishments as a Special Olympian. The Junior Achievement organization renovated a former car dealership catty-corner to us and across the street a former sewing factory was transformed into a technology building and now houses employees for the company that bought the Pfaltzgraff Pottery Company.

As I was changing physically, emotionally, spiritually and intellectually so was the neighboring area around 515 South George Street.

The Byrnes HEC was not the reason for all this positive change but it was a critical component. Since 1995, the community began to stream into the 500 block of South George; expectant mothers going to the Mother/Child Clinic, 5th graders attending Exchange

City to learn about the business of running a community, and bus load after bus load of eager students coming to the Byrnes Health Education Center to learn about the wonders of life.

Over the past nineteen years, the health of our community has evolved as well. In 1994, the Healthy York County Coalition was created to bring the community together to improve the quality of life for everyone. The York City Health Bureau works tirelessly to improve the health of the 44,000 city residents and keeps the health statistics on the 300,000 York County individuals. Heart disease, cancer and diabetes were the top three notorious killers in our community. However, in a recent Health Bureau Report, it was noted that "over the past ten years the number of deaths from heart disease, and cancer was declining. Education efforts by the Bureau of Health and other local/national organizations, as well as technological advances in treating disease contribute to this trend." We are playing our small part.

The Center for Traffic Safety reported that the percentage of the total number of vehicle deaths due to alcohol over the past ten years had dropped from 50 percent to 33 percent. In addition, the number of alcohol related crashes had gone down by 20 percent. This was due to the combined efforts of everyone; state police sobriety tests, the Center for Traffic Safety and education by schools and the Byrnes Health Education Center.

How much of a role has the Byrnes HEC played in the reduction of preventable deaths in our community? In my heart and soul I know that we have made a difference. Collecting quantitative research indicating whether or not attendance in our educational programs creates lasting change is difficult. We have hundreds of personal accounts of individuals who say they have made healthy choices after participating in our programs.

Several weeks ago, I received an email from one of our health educators. The subject line read: "we are changing lives." She proceeded to write about how she had been asked to come to the Substance Abuse Teaching Theater to show some of our exhibits on smoking. She left her overflowing desk and went to the lobby to greet two females: a daughter and her mother.

They had come from a clinic appointment in an adjacent building. The daughter remembered being in our teaching theaters through her school visits and wanted her mother to see the exhibits on tobacco. She was worried about her mother because she smoked and wanted her to see the horrible damage that tobacco does to lungs.

(*Did you know* that each lung contains 300 million microscopic alveoli, tiny air sacs that exchange oxygen and carbon dioxide for our bodies? When the 200 degree tobacco smoke is forced into them they begin to rupture... never to be regenerated.)

As our educator explained that one cigarette contains over 4,000 chemicals and displayed a slide of a blackened, cancerous lung, tears began to run down the mother's face. She sobbed, "I did not know that this is what I was doing to my lungs. I want to stop smoking." The health educator was amazed that once again her knowledge and our dramatic displays of a healthy and unhealthy respiratory system could so effectively demonstrate the power of prevention and encourage healthy choices. She walked the mother and daughter to our front desk and gave them information where the mother could seek help to quit smoking.

PASSION CAN CHANGE YOUR COMMUNITY

Up until now I've been telling you about my quest to start the Byrnes HEC, how my dream-come-true has changed me and the effects it has had on my hometown, York, Pennsylvania. Now, after nineteen years of educating people to make healthy choices, there is an additional part of my dream that I would like to see happen; I want to inspire others to put their passion into action, become involved in their communities and make their community part of who they are!

PASSION... SMALL ACTS OF KINDNESS

I'd like you to take a moment and reflect on your life. Think about all the people that you have touched: friends, neighbors, church members and even perhaps, complete strangers. Remember,

Jimmie Stewart as George Bailey in the movie, "It's A Wonderful Life?" Clarence, his "angel", had to show George that his giving to others truly made a difference in his home town. During the Depression, George Bailey lent his bank's money to one and all. When George later found himself in need of the same compassion and help to keep his bank open his numerous small acts of kindness were returned to him by those same people. He truly was the "richest man in town." Kindness does not remain stationary or even go away: it moves. It finds another place to manifest itself. We are the vehicles for kindness to move from one person to another.

How much more could you do for others? Let me share a personal story about how a single letter made an amazing difference.

One bright, beautiful winter day in January, 2000, a young woman waited in anticipation on the Wrightsville (York County) side of the Susquehanna River. Today, she would meet for the first time a male college student that she had been corresponding with for several months through the internet. Tragedy was about to overshadow this first innocent encounter.

Unbeknownst to them, as these two college students were walking and getting acquainted a man was stalking them. He had been driving slowly behind the couple in his pickup truck. Suddenly, he startled them by waving his shotgun and demanding that the woman get in the front seat while he tied the young man to his dog in the bay of the truck. He raped the young woman, drove them to the edge of the river, ordered them into the icy water, shot each of them several times and left them for dead.

A short time later, some fishermen discovered these two young people floating near the river's edge and called 911. They were rushed to the hospital's Emergency Department and then into surgery.

As I read of this horrific tragedy in our local newspaper I immediately thought: what are the families of these victims going to think of my hometown? What could our community do to show these victims and their families that we were appalled by their tragedy and we cared about their recovery?

So, I wrote a Letter to the Editor of a local newspaper and suggested a CAMPAIGN FOR COMPASSION. The response was an overwhelming community outpouring of love: flowers, cards, teddy bears, candy, free lodging at our historic downtown hotel for the families, and certificates for meals began to arrive in their hospital rooms. In addition, the police worked diligently to locate and imprison the man responsible for this horrible crime.

Several weeks after the tragedy, with a tremendous feeling of pride in my heart, I wrote a thank you letter to my community for their generous giving to these victims and their families. Everyone wanted to do something to share their concern and compassion. The letter to the editor simply activated their caring.

Below are both letters.

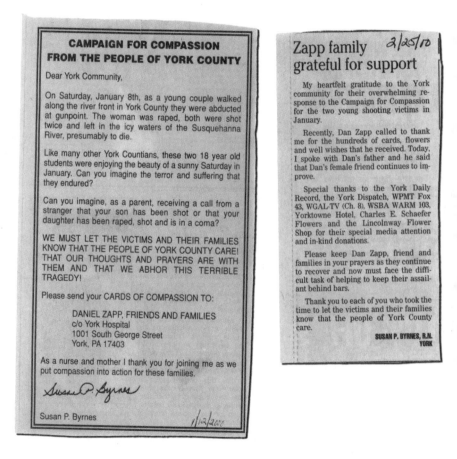

CAMPAIGN FOR COMPASSION FROM THE PEOPLE OF YORK COUNTY

Dear York Community,

On Saturday, January 8th, as a young couple walked along the river front in York County they were abducted at gunpoint. The woman was raped, both were shot twice and left in the icy waters of the Susquehanna River, presumably to die.

Like many other York Countians, these two 18 year old students were enjoying the beauty of a sunny Saturday in January. Can you imagine the terror and suffering that they endured?

Can you imagine, as a parent, receiving a call from a stranger that your son has been shot or that your daughter has been raped, shot and is in a coma?

WE MUST LET THE VICTIMS AND THEIR FAMILIES KNOW THAT THE PEOPLE OF YORK COUNTY CARE! THAT OUR THOUGHTS AND PRAYERS ARE WITH THEM AND THAT WE ABHOR THIS TERRIBLE TRAGEDY!

Please send your CARDS OF COMPASSION TO:

DANIEL ZAPP, FRIENDS AND FAMILIES
c/o York Hospital
1001 South George Street
York, PA 17403

As a nurse and mother I thank you for joining me as we put compassion into action for these families.

Susan P. Byrnes

Susan P. Byrnes

1/12/2010

Zapp family grateful for support 2/25/10

My heartfelt gratitude to the York community for their overwhelming response to the Campaign for Compassion for the two young shooting victims in January.

Recently, Dan Zapp called to thank me for the hundreds of cards, flowers and well wishes that he received. Today, I spoke with Dan's father and he said that Dan's female friend continues to improve.

Special thanks to the York Daily Record, the York Dispatch, WPMT Fox 43, WGAL-TV (Ch. 8), WSBA WARM 103, Yorktowne Hotel, Charles E. Schaefer Flowers and the Lincolnway Flower Shop for their special media attention and in-kind donations.

Please keep Dan Zapp, friend and families in your prayers as they continue to recover and now must face the difficult task of helping to keep their assailant behind bars.

Thank you to each of you who took the time to let the victims and their families know that the people of York County care.

SUSAN P. BYRNES, R.N.
YORK

7

Reflections On Giving

It's been said that, everything changes after a gift is given: neither the giver, nor the receiver is ever the same again. My nineteen years of building and gathering gifts for the Byrnes HEC have taught me that this is very true. In this chapter, I'd like to share with you some of my thoughts, reflections, experiences and wonderful memories having to do with giving and receiving. Hopefully, these stories will inspire you to give and receive.

One thing I've learned is that all giving makes a difference. Sometimes giving is very easy; writing a check to a favorite non-profit or disaster appeal, putting your envelope in the church's offering basket or buying lemonade from a child's roadside stand. I remember two glorious times when receiving this kind of gift made a huge difference in the building of my dream.

CAPITAL CAMPAIGN SURPRISE

It was the end of another hot, humid summer day in our eleventh month of daily asking people for money. I was ready to check-in with my three teenagers when I heard the unmistakable creaking of the stairs leading to our rent-free, second floor offices at The BYRNES Group. A handsome gentleman turned the corner and tentatively entered my rather simple surroundings. He congratulated me on the mission of the health education center. We had not met and as I expressed my thanks for his kind remarks and was about to ask how he knew of us he handed a check for $2,500 to me and said, "Keep up the good work". I broke into a huge smile and embraced him. Clearly, he was embarrassed by my enthusiastic response to his generosity. His check took us over the two million dollar capital campaign goal. The memories of all the hours of solicitations by so many dedicated volunteers washed over me. This one person with a single check symbolized all the efforts that comprise a year-long community fund drive. I will never forget the power of that moment.

YOU JUST NEVER KNOW

During our capital campaign, Randy and I made a number of major gift calls together. He later said the only reason I invited him was so that I did not have to drive. (I didn't realize he knew that at the time.) At one of our meetings, with a current Byrnes HEC board member, we discussed what turned out to be a very successful and significant pledge commitment. As we concluded the meeting the board member chuckled and stated that we should go immediately to the office of one of his close colleagues and carry the challenge that this compatriot should match his pledge or forever live with the fact that he would walk in his shadow. His sheepish grin and twinkling eyes were evidence that he was feeling very satisfied with his cleverness.

Randy and I practically injured ourselves in our haste to carry this challenging message to his unsuspecting friend. The second party responded like we all knew he would and the Health Education Center was the double beneficiary. These are the corporate leaders who financially sustain the organizations so vital to our community.

It was wonderful to be the recipient of these fund raising gifts that lessened our financial challenges. Several months later, I had an opportunity to "pass it along."

One rainy, dark, winter evening, I followed my Dad's advice to open my heart and wallet at the same time. I should have been home by now making dinner but I had to stop at the drug store for a prescription for one of our children. I was patiently waiting in line. The young woman in front of me was clearly distressed when the cashier told her the cost for the prescription. She said, "Oh, no, it can't be that much. My daughter has an ear infection and she is in so much pain and I don't have that much money." As I overheard this conversation my heart did a flip-flop. What if I didn't have money to pay for my child's prescription? I quickly opened my wallet and handed her a twenty dollar bill. At first she refused, and then with tears in her eyes she said thank you. I do not even know this woman's name, and yet, I remembered this simple, spontaneous act of giving so long ago, and still feel warm and happy about it.

UP CLOSE AND PERSONAL

It seems to me a greater level of contributing to your community involves thoughtful giving, which takes more of your own time. I think that my Dad is a perfect example.

Every month, for the past six years, Charlie Petron, who lives on a fixed income, walks through the bright red doors of 515 South George Street to hand-deliver his personal check to support the Byrnes HEC. He drives by our facility, three days a week, on his way to work and delights in the fact that he can save a stamp by dropping off his check. He also declines a thank you note so we can save an additional thirty-nine cents. His current giving is over one year ahead of his generous annual pledge to our HeartBeat Scholarship Program. I have learned from a MASTER GIVER OF MODEST MEANS.

Some people might be embarrassed by only being able to give a little but Cardinal Cushing once said, "Never measure your generosity by what you give, but rather, by what you have left."

(*Did you know* that in 2005, Americans gave over two billion dollars to non-profits and that eighty percent of the givers were individuals?)

LEARNING TO GIVE

Even having such wonderful role models as my parents, I have to admit, I wasn't always a giver. When Randy and I were first married we received a packet of weekly envelopes from the church and I responded by saying, "I can't believe that they expect us to support them when we are trying to raise a family." Then I remembered my Dad filling our family's church envelopes with money (in spite of a salesman's salary and seven children) and how my six brothers and sisters and I also had to put part of our weekly allowance in the kids' envelopes.

Randy and I began to give to our church and gradually learned to give to our community both personally and through Randy's business. The more we gave, the more we wanted to give and I believe the more we received. It is an amazing circle.

Teaching the mechanics of giving to children can begin at a young age. Children learn by watching their parents give of their time, talent and treasure to their community. In addition, some schools require that students give back by performing service hours or building something for their community. Susan Crites Price of the Council on Foundations' Family Foundation Services staff, has written a common sense book, The Giving Family. You may order the book at www.thegiving family.org.

Learning to Give (www.learningtogive.org) is a K-12 project of the Council of Michigan Foundations. Their mission is to educate youth about philanthropy, the nonprofit sector and volunteerism. Families can join together when giving to their communities; feeding the hungry, raising money through a walk for their favorite charity, or learning how to effectively recycle and reduce our waste products. Children can reap the joys of giving also.

What if everyone who felt that they have more than they needed gave the excess to others?

CIRCLE OF GIVING

Sometimes, you have the special opportunity to complete the circle of giving. You give a gift to an organization and receive a thank you, you continue to give and become part of the mission and vision, all the while reaping the joy of giving.

Have you experienced this circle of giving? I hope so... it is amazingly enriching to life. Fortunately, I have. People have given their time, talent and money to build the health education center and improve the health of our community. I received these gifts to build the health education center. In return, my life has been blessed with an incredible amount of loving relationships.

Relationships are the core of all gift-giving decisions both large and small. While individuals may donate large amounts of wealth to institutions, churches, schools or local non-profit organizations

I believe at the root of their generosity is a relationship that impacted them in a special way. I have selected the following stories, with the permission of the givers, to highlight a few who have given to their community to make things happen. These two experiences are just a few of the many mystical, magical moments in the creation of my dream.

My loving relationship with Mildred S. Gabrielson (Milly) began seventeen years ago. A board member mentioned to me that he had a client who was a retired school teacher who loved children and education. My super angel Milly has a generous heart and a deep love of education. I called Milly. We arranged to have lunch and hit it off immediately. Together, we traveled to 515 South George Street. We carefully walked around oil patches and discarded car parts that littered the 30,000 square foot newly acquired building.

Milly quickly became part of the Byrnes HEC family. Throughout my seven year pregnancy she was by my side; cheering, encouraging and supporting my "baby" financially. We have become kindred spirits. We know all about one another's family through pictures and stories during hundreds of lunches at little sandwich shops and country clubs.

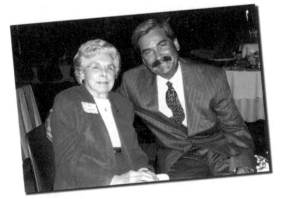

Milly Gabrielson and long-time board member, Jim Bergdoll

My dream of keeping my community healthy became Milly's dream. She has given her time, talent and treasure to build a leading resource for quality health education programs. After generously participating in our capital campaign, she established two permanent funds to endow her annual gift to our HeartBeat Scholarship Program. The Mildred S. Gabrielson Body Shop for

Young Learners became a reality when she gave a major gift for new exhibits to benefit our youngest learners in kindergarten and first grade. (Milly's room is actually in the former paint shop area of the car dealership.) And the ultimate gift, Milly is leaving her legacy through a bequest to endow a chair for our Director of Youth Education. At the dedication ceremony, Milly said "I had the same idea about children and the importance of teaching them to be healthy as Susie did."

Over and over, Milly has shared with me how joyful she is because of her giving to the Byrnes HEC. She says that she feels so good knowing that she is helping so many children. Milly spreads this joy with her friends and many of them now support us. Milly is an excellent example of reaping the joy of giving while you are living. Milly will be ninety-six years young in May, 2007.

Before Milly and I say good-bye, we always say "I love you" to one another. Loving relationships are the icing on the cake when you give back to your community.

Several years ago at Christmas time, the Byrnes Health Education Center received a $100 check from a local bank's trust office. This was a new gift so I called the trust officer. She explained that she was familiar with us (Sam Bressi was her son's soccer coach) and she had encouraged her client to send a check to us. I asked if I could call the giver to express my gratitude. She said sure. I made the call to James M. Henderson, Jr. "Jimmie", (I'm one of the few who is allowed to call him by this special name) has lived alone in his boyhood home since his mother died many years ago. He was thrilled to hear from me. During our conversation, I learned that as a young boy he had contracted encephalitis, a life threatening illness, that damaged his brain and nervous system. As Jimmie has aged, his nervous system has deteriorated.

He lives with tremors in his hands and braces on both ankles to support his legs when he walks. These disabilities do not hinder Jimmie's ability to travel to his favorite charities many times a week. My initial call to Jimmie was the first of hundreds. Just like Milly, we shared family stories and pictures. I practiced my Christmas carols so I could play them for him on his lovely grand piano.

We both had tears in our eyes after my novice performance. Our birthdays are one day apart so I take his favorite coconut cake to him every year. We also share a love of gardening. Because Jimmie can't get down and dig in his mother's beloved flower beds, I do. I weed, plant geraniums and assist the gardening service to make Jimmie's gardens beautiful. It is absolutely wonderful to see the joy on his face as he looks out the window at his gorgeous flowers.

Jimmie gives to many local and national organizations. He told me that he has decided to direct most of his giving to our community. He says that it makes him feel so good to give. He often tells me how much he treasures our friendship. Because I am a nurse he can share some of his frustrations with his health challenges and he knows that I appreciate his trials. My weekly calls and bimonthly visits seem to bring some sunshine into his life. In addition, a bubbly staff member has also befriended Jimmie and he calls her his breath of fresh air.

Jimmie, along with one of his devoted care-givers, came to see the Byrnes HEC. He loved our dynamic exhibits and the 88 colors in our renovated building. Recently, he asked if he could stop in more often. My response was, "of course" so we arranged to have our staff meet Jimmie. He wanted to be included as part of the Byrnes HEC family and we welcomed this angel with open arms.

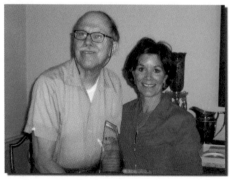

James Henderson receiving an award from me

On a weekly basis, Jimmie asks what he can do for us. We always have an answer; flowers for our annual meeting, office supplies, hand-held exhibits, major annual gifts and he also has remembered the Byrnes HEC in his will.

(*Did you know* that 80% of individuals give to charity during their lifetime, but less than ten percent remember these charities in their wills. Have you remembered your charities in your will?)

Recently, I asked Jimmie why he gives so much to so many. He said, "Because it gives ME a feeling of peace. People really need support even if you can only give a little. My parents felt the same way. I was taught to give as a teenager through their example."

Jimmie, like Milly, is reaping the joys of giving while he is living and the Byrnes HEC is deeply grateful for his generosity.

Other ways to GIVE…Comfort and Kindness

Giving doesn't always have to involve money. Giving from the heart connects people to people and gives hope to one another. Hope strengthens the heart and despair ravages it. According to a study published in August 1997 in the American Heart Association's Journal, hopelessness speeds up the narrowing of the arteries. Giving from the heart, on the other hand, heals the body and soul, even in times of trouble and sorrow. I know this to be true from a personal experience.

The Sunday after 9/11/01 our church was packed. People wanted to be surrounded with familiar faces and reassured by their presence. I know that I did. My husband was out of town and the U. S. Marines had called three times trying to contact our son and call him to active duty. Instead of healing our hearts, the priest chose to emphasize the negative part of this tragedy with stories of torture and murder that had occurred in the church's history. As I gazed around the church I caught the look of despair in people's eyes. We needed to be comforted rather than listen to negative thoughts. I felt that I needed to do something uplifting and I responded as a nurse to help those in need. I rose from my seat…

I began the long walk to the altar thinking maybe I could find the right words to reassure and comfort. I whispered in the priest's ear that I would like to address the congregation. He looked shocked, staring at me as if I were a ghost, but nodded ok. I could feel my heart pounding. But surprisingly, when I opened my mouth the words started to pour forth from my heart. I acknowledged the 9/11 tragedy and how each of us was grieving even though many of us did not know the victims personally. We all wanted to do something positive. I told them a story of how a car mechanic had helped an employee of the Byrnes HEC this past week. He had given money to her so she could take a cab back to work while her car was being serviced. He gave cheerfully, without asking or wanting to be reimbursed. I challenged the congregation to do as this mechanic had done; give of themselves to someone everyday that week whether it was a family member, friend, or complete stranger. Nothing would alleviate the sorrow and grief of the 9/11 tragedy but people giving to people, practicing random acts of kindness, would reaffirm and deepen our human spirit which connects us all.

As I walked back to my pew people began to applaud. I knew that many lives would experience the kindness of another in the days to follow. Everyone understood the need to reach out and assure another person that they were not alone: acts of thoughtfulness and caring help heal our sorrow and lift our souls.

GIVING from the HEART
Prologue

Life is a gift.

We do not know how long this precious gift will last.

As a mother and daughter-in-law, I continue to grieve for our family's loss of Mom-Mom. As my children, nieces and nephews have graduated from high school and college, as we have celebrated the joyous occasions of three weddings, (one daughter and two nieces), my heart aches because Mom-Mom, who loved her six precious grandchildren (she never got to meet two additional grandsons), and a good party, was not with us. Sometimes I wonder…if she could have stopped smoking and only drank in moderation would she be with us today?

I see the results of unhealthy lifestyles everywhere. And yet, through research and education, we now know how the body works and what we need to do to keep it working well.

So, what stops us from MAKING HEALTHY CHOICES?

Admittedly, not all diseases can be prevented. But the biggest killers in this country, heart disease and related factors of obesity and diabetes as well as some cancers especially those caused by tobacco could be greatly reduced if people would only change their behavior. ONE SMALL STEP AT A TIME. Loving ourselves enough to make healthy choices; walking instead of taking elevators, choosing frozen yogurt instead of ice cream, turning off the TV and going outside to garden, walking or playing with our children, grandchildren, or neighborhood kids.

My wish for all precious children is that prevention would become a national priority. **We must invest billions into keeping people well instead of spending trillions to treat disease**.

Healthcare professionals, government, businesses, and families must partner and focus on HEALTHY LIFESTYLE CHOICES. We must reduce the number of overweight children in our country, currently one in three (according to the National Center for Health Statistics), and the number of children who smoke their first cigarette each day, 3,000.

4.5 MILLION CHILDREN AND TEENAGERS SMOKE IN THE U.S.

Tobacco companies spend approximately **$15,000,000,000 A YEAR** to **addict our children.** (Campaign for Tobacco Free Kids)

450,000 PEOPLE DIE EACH YEAR FROM TOBACCO PRODUCTS. MOST OF THESE DEATHS ARE PREVENTABLE!

We must TAKE CHARGE OF OUR HEALTH and MAKE HEALTHY CHOICES starting today.

Twelve years ago in the fall of 1995, in a speech to the York community, C. Everett Koop, M.D. stated emphatically, the biggest influence on the health of our nation is not on advanced technology, it is individuals taking charge of their health and being a partner in their healthcare.

Have you done this? What would make you TAKE CHARGE OF YOUR HEALTH?

If creating the Susan P. Byrnes Health Education Center prevented one child from lighting his first cigarette, inspired one parent to cook healthy food for his/her family, or motivated one overweight forty-year-old to lose 20 pounds, then all my years of volunteering and investing my time, talent and treasure was worth every minute.

The greatest sacrifice for me was the time that I took away from my children and husband. As the weeks began to fly by after I had presided over my last board meeting in September, 2002, I began to experience my body relaxing and my mind and heart reflecting on the past fourteen years. An overwhelming feeling of missing the growing-up years of my children weighed heavily on my heart. So, I composed a letter to them that I planned to read on Christmas Eve.

In the letter, I shared my great pride in whom they had become; our teacher (Katie), college student (Kristy), and U.S. Marine, (Dan). They had grown into caring, self-reliant and hard-working young adults. This pride was offset however by a mother's guilt that consumed me with questions of what had they sacrificed on my behalf? All the hours away from home at meetings, tired and irritable at times when I had placed my Byrnes HEC priorities above theirs, were now haunting me. With a shaky voice and tears streaming down my face, I asked for their forgiveness for giving so much of myself to the Byrnes HEC. I thanked them and Randy for helping me to build my dream for York.

One by one they told me stories of their lives during their teenage years; memories that were meaningful for them but had passed before me like so many events during that time. Each of them had wonderful vignettes and tales that caused us to laugh and cry into the evening. They were unanimous in their conviction that they had not been shortchanged but were so proud of me and the Susan P. Byrnes Health Education Center. What an incredible gift.

In the two years that it has taken to compose this book I have had the deep pleasure (most of the time) of reliving the creation of the Susan P. Byrnes Health Education Center. I have written this book to HONOR EVERYONE AND ANYONE who assisted with my dream come true. They have a special place in my heart.

I encourage each of you to dream your own dreams. Put your passion into action. Give to as many people as you can for as long as you can. Believe in the power of one.

YOU CAN MAKE A DIFFERENCE!

Are you serious about creating your own not-for-profit or learning more about gathering financial gifts to improve the quality of life for others? If so, the next two appendices are for you.

The third appendix is for those of you who would like to establish a health education center in your hometown.

Using my personal experiences, I have organized my thoughts into two areas: The HeART of Gift Gathering and Building Your Dream.

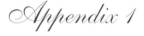

Appendix 1

THE HeART OF GIFT GATHERING

(Did you know: that your heart is going to beat 100,000 times today? It is a small muscle that weighs less than one pound. It pumps blood through 60,000 miles of blood vessels every minute of every hour of every day.)

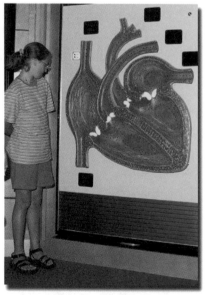

Fund raising or gift gathering is the HEART of any organization. Every gift pumps money into every aspect of your organization. It is critical that **you give first** before you ask anyone to invest in your mission and vision. You want to be able to say to potential givers, "will you join me?"

For nineteen years I have been volunteering my time to gather gifts for the Byrnes

Our five foot heart

Health Education Center. And yes, I am a giver. This act of giving keeps me well and releases endorphins in my brain. The chemical reaction makes the body feel good.

Research has demonstrated that giving of yourself can actually lower stress, strengthen the immune system, and make your heart stronger. Have you experienced the joy and health benefits of giving? It's fun. It's easy.

THREE STEPS TO BECOME A GIVER

love yourself
believe in the power of one
develop PMA-Positive Mental Attitude

#1 YOU must **love yourself** enough to take charge of your health. You can be all that you dream if you have a strong mind, body and spirit. Balance your home, work and play. Make a commitment to get some exercise every day; walk around your yard, take the stairs instead of the elevator, get up from your desk at lunchtime and walk to a restaurant for lunch. Make healthier food choices. Join a yoga class. Take a walk and murmur out-loud the first five things for which you are most grateful. I guarantee that if you feel well, you will begin to think about giving to others, you will develop peace of mind and you will LIVE WELL.

#2 YOU can make a difference. You must **believe that one person** can make a difference. (Read the book Power of One by Bryce Courtney.) Use your "gifts" to make a difference. Can you sing? Join a community group of singers that sing at Christmas in hospitals and nursing homes. Are you a good listener? Volunteer at an assisted living facility to play games and interact with the residents. Do you like to drive? Call your Area Agency on Aging and see if you can do errands for an elderly person. Get involved in your community. Read your local paper, identify community organizations that appeal to you, call them and ask to get involved. Most organizations can use volunteers.

#3 YOU can **develop PMA**-Positive Mental Attitude. Remember Pollyanna and her GLAD GAME that her missionary Dad taught to her? Her Dad was a minister and they were in a poor country but he taught Pollyanna that when she was feeling homesick or blue to think about what made her glad; the clean water that she could drink, the beautiful flowers and the love of her mother and father. Everyone gets down in the dumps. Everyone can be glad about something and adjust his/her attitude. Try this, for one day smile at everyone you meet. Most people will return your smile even if it takes a few seconds. Most of us should be giving thanks for a lot of our blessings. Make a list. Keep it on your desk and when you are feeling blue, read the list out loud and recharge your PMA.

Now, that you love yourself, believe in your power, have your PMA, and are a giver, you are ready to begin asking people to join you in giving.

LOVE YOURSELF WITH KINDNESS. Pope John XXIII

To quote David Rockefeller: 'never apologize for asking for money for a worthy cause'.

MY THREE SECRETS FOR GIFT GATHERING:

PASSION
PERSISTENCE
PATIENCE

PASSION

People give to people. And they give to enthusiastic people - passionate people who believe in the mission of their organization. When I was gathering gifts for our capital campaign, I knew that there were many "doubting Thomases." Why does York need another not-for-profit? Why do kids need to know about their bodies? This is a huge undertaking by one petite nurse. But these same individuals gave large amounts of money because they felt my enthusiasm and passion. They could not say no. How could they disappoint me? After all, educating children to make healthy decisions is fundamental to a child's well-being.

Recruit passionate ambassadors and board members. It is critical to get the right people asking the right people for large gifts. Identify the movers and shakers in your community, get them excited about your idea/organization and then ask them to initiate some of your larger gift gathering.

PERSISTENCE

Persistence prevails when all else fails. This quote by Calvin Coolidge has been on my desk for 19 years. When I would be in the midst of a particularly discouraging phone call, I would repeat this over and over in my mind.   Never take the first "no." **Reword, rework, revisit**. Get potential givers to experience your organization. It will sell itself.

I ask people to give money so children and their families can be taught about their magnificent bodies and how to keep them working throughout their lifetime. It is thrilling. There is no better gift than having good health. When I ask people for money I'm helping them to be well.

Grassroots gift gathering and treating givers as I would like to be treated has been my mantra. Has it been hard work? Has it been rewarding? Yes and Yes. When you are passionate about your organization and when you are also a giver, people will give and many times they will be generous.

PATIENCE

In order to grow gifts you must be a good gardener. You plant a seed with a giver, you water it with attention, information and companionship. After many months and years, you may have the potential for a beautiful blossoming of a major gift or bequest. You must be patient, never forceful with your desires or wishes but you must, on occasion, make the ask. Ask givers to endow their annual gift, or ask for a major need or ask that they remember the organization in their will. If you don't have the courage and conviction to look someone in the eye and ask them for a gift for your organization how can you expect to receive a gift from them?

GUIDELINES FOR GIFT GATHERING

Hear - do you hear what I hear?

> My first question when I make a call; "Is this a good time for you to talk?"
> Are you truly HERE when you are with your givers? Do you truly listen?

Enthusiasm - ya gotta believe
Passion is contagious.

Accurate - it's in the details
Excellent record keeping and always truthful.

Relationship - the 'Golden Rule'
Treat your givers as you would like to be treated

Thank you - "No really, Thank you"
Again and again, thank your givers

In conclusion I would like to remind you that everyone who walks through your door or calls on the phone could be "the millionaire next door." Treat everyone the same; with dignity and respect. They could be your next major giver.

The following story came to me over the internet. While Harvard denies that this scenario occurred, the moral of the tale is profound.

A lady in a faded gingham dress and her husband, dressed in a homespun threadbare suit, stepped off the train in Boston, and walked timidly without an appointment into the outer office of the President of Harvard University.

"We want to see the president," the man said softly.

"He'll be busy all day," the secretary snapped.

"We'll wait," the lady replied.

For hours, the secretary ignored them, hoping that the couple would finally become discouraged and go away. They didn't. And the secretary grew frustrated and finally decided to disturb the president, even though it was a chore she always regretted to do.

"Maybe if they just see you for a few minutes, they'll leave," she told him. And he sighed in exasperation and nodded.

Someone of his importance obviously didn't have the time to spend with them, but he detested gingham dresses and homespun suits cluttering up his outer office.

The president, stern-faced with dignity, strutted toward the couple. The lady told him, "We had a son that attended Harvard for one year. He loved Harvard. He was happy here. But about a year ago, he was accidentally killed. And my husband and I would like to erect a memorial to him, somewhere on campus.

The president wasn't touched; he was shocked. "Madame," he said gruffly, "We can't put up a statue for every person who attended Harvard and died. If we did, this place would look like a cemetery."

"Oh, no," the lady explained quickly, "We don't want to erect a statue. We thought we would like to give a building to Harvard.

The president rolled his eyes. He glanced at the gingham dress and homespun suit, and then exclaimed, "A building! Do you have any earthly idea how much a building costs? We have over seven and a half million dollars in the physical plant at Harvard." For a moment the lady was silent. The president was pleased. He could get rid of them now.

The lady turned to her husband and said quietly, "Is that all it costs to start a University? Why don't we just start our own?" Her husband nodded.

The president's face wilted in confusion and bewilderment as Mr. and Mrs. Leland Stanford walked away, traveling to Palo Alto, California, where in 1885 they established Stanford University, as a memorial to their son about whom Harvard no longer cared.

You know what happens when you ASSUME something.... Don't let this arrogance happen to you and your organization.

Appendix 2

BUILDING YOUR DREAM

DON'T EXPECT LIFE TO BE WORTH LIVING, MAKE IT THAT WAY.

ANONYMOUS

Many people have asked me; how did I start a not-for-profit organization. My answer: one small step at a time.

Remember, I'm a nurse. I was an organizer and a great cheerleader but had never started my own business. Nor was I business savvy so I had to surround myself with individuals who possessed the skills that I lacked. And, believe me, there were many. But I was passionate about my mission and I was volunteering my time. For these two reasons, people patiently listened as I explained my dream of a health education center for our community. How could they say no to someone who was committed enough to work for free?

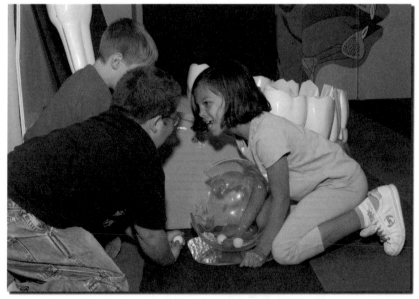

Dental health fun

FOLLOW THESE STEPS TO SUCCESS:

- Research and meet others who are involved in like-ventures
- Establish a Board of Directors: look for the three W's: Work, Wisdom, Wealth; don't settle for less than one W
- Create a Mission and Vision: keep it simple and short
- Make presentations to whomever will stand still for 5 minutes
- Obtain testimonial letters of support
- Design brochures, newsletters and a database
- Gather financial gifts: begin with board members, businesses, service organizations, individuals, local grants
- Hire an entrepreneurial CEO/President
- Establish a working partnership between staff and board
- Plan your work and work your plan.. do strategic planning
- Balance your budget from day one
- Know when it is time to step aside as leader
- Recognize the angels that appear and assist you
- HAVE FUN

When I began researching and visiting health education centers in March, 1988, I really did not know how long nor how difficult the process was going to be. I began to give presentations in my home during the day, before my children came home from school and then in the evenings when Randy could be with the kids and put them to bed.

As I met with people, I would decide if they possessed the three W's necessary to be a successful board member: WEALTH, WISDOM AND WORK. As I began to gather board members, I would ask them for the names of three other people that they thought should know about my dream.

NETWORKING IS CRUCIAL TO YOUR SUCCESS

I always sent personal thank you notes to every person that I met.

When we reached five board members we began to hold monthly board meetings. These meetings were so important because it made me realize that the buck stopped with me. I had to make progress and report it to the Board. Roberts Rules of Order are a must even for small business meetings. Start and end your meetings on time!

Our board meetings have always been graced with my homemade chocolate chip cookies...terrific enticement for board attendance.

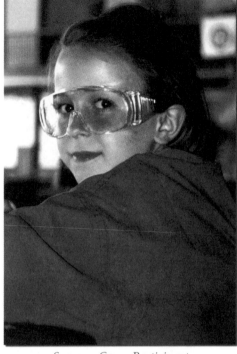

Summer Camp Participant

Begin your database as soon as you start to meet with people and regularly update it. Then start a one page newsletter and send it to these individuals every other month. You need to keep your dream in front of as many people as possible. Meet with the editors of local and regional newspapers as well as the TV stations. Ask them for in-kind space/ads. Get on free TV and community radio shows and pitch your organization again and again. Ask a local printer to print an in-kind simple brochure. Carry them in your trunk and leave them in your doctor, dentist, attorney, and accountant's office. Visit your minister or pastor and ask to speak at your church or synagogue. Gather your friends in your home; serve homemade food with your ideas for making the world a better place.

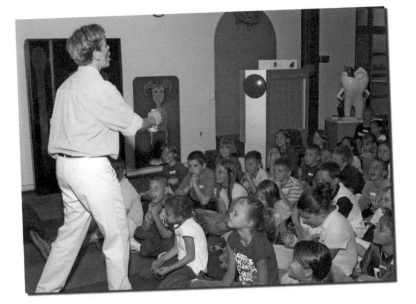

PUBLICIZE YOUR DREAM EVERY DAY AS OFTEN AS YOU CAN.

My gift gathering career, aka, fund-raising, began when I asked the Young Women's Club of York for a $500 grant to rent a bus to take the Medical Alliance Members to Easton, PA to see the Weller Health Education Center. I was successful and have been picking pockets with affection for 19 years: from friends and family, corporations, hospitals, service organizations and local, state and federal government. Sure it's hard but a ton of FUN. I have met hundreds of caring, giving individuals and only a few, not-so-giving. Some of my closest friends are my "partners" in the fund-raising arena.

FUND-RAISING IS CRITICAL TO YOUR FINANCIAL STABILITY

YEP, YOU GUESSED IT, CHOCOLATE CHIP COOKIES TO GIVERS TOO.

As you follow your steps to success remember to accept advice, encouragement and sometimes special assistance from "angels." During the creation of my dream, I developed an inner and outer circle of supporters. My inner circle was led by my husband, Randy, my extended family and beloved board members and staff. The outer circle consisted of individuals in the region and occasionally nationally recognized celebrities who encouraged and inspired me with their kindness. Remember, the Father of Prevention, C. Everett Koop, MD? After ten years of correspondence with me, he now signs his letters, Chick. His closest friends gave him that nickname.

Katharine Houghton Hepburn began sending notes to me in 1989.

One of my favorite Sunday morning activities used to be reading *Parade Magazine* that was part of our local paper. I loved reading the inspirational articles about people who made a difference in our world. (I secretly hope that one day there will be an article about the Byrnes Health Educational Center.) In 1989, I read a glorious article about Katharine Hepburn, in honor of her 80th birthday. She had agreed to be photographed with a huge bouquet of flowers. I read about her father who had been an urologist and her mother who had raised three children and found the time to be an activist for women's rights. And so, I thought, because of Ms. Hepburn's feisty spirit and keen mind she might like the idea of my dream for my hometown. That evening, after I had put the children to bed, I poured out my heart and soul to Ms. Hepburn in a letter. Never, did I imagine that I would hear from this famous woman.

Several weeks passed. As I was sorting our mail one evening, a little white envelope with a New York City postmark caught my attention. I was stunned as I opened it and saw in simple red block letters: KATHARINE HOUGHTON HEPBURN at the top of the note paper. It was type-written with simple sentences that stated: ***Thank you for your letter. I think what you are doing is wildly important. Good for you and good luck.*** signed ***K. Hepburn.***

I ran from my office to our family room to share this fabulous note with my husband, Randy. A big smile crossed his lips. This little nurse from Spry received a letter from Katharine Hepburn. I immediately went back to my office and wrote a thank you note and updated her on my progress with the Health Education Center.

This correspondence continued for many years. I have eight notes from Ms. Hepburn. I learned that she was a tennis player, as I was, but we never got a chance to play together. I spoke with her assistant on several occasions. (Did you know that Ms. Hepburn took her own trash to the curb when she lived in the Turtle Bay area of NYC?)

Ms. Hepburn was unable to attend our grand opening in 1995 but she sent me a congratulatory note.

Why am I sharing these stories? Because I want you to realize that when you follow your heart and build your dream, sometimes you meet a few stars. Perhaps, your life will even be gifted with real-life angels who will shine brightly in your corner. Dreams are never achieved alone.

So, take that first step and begin your dream. You never know who your angels will be.

Katharine Houghton Hepburn

III - 16 - 1995

Dear Susie Byrnes -
        Good for you - I'm sorry but I
cannot join you on April 29th and
30th - Continued good luck for your
project -
        Katharine Hepburn

Appendix 3

The Susan P. Byrnes Health and Education Center (Byrnes HEC), and the National Association of Health Education Centers, (NAHEC)

The Susan P. Byrnes Health Education Center was incorporated in March, 1989.

Mission: To educate and inspire people of all ages to make healthy choices.

Vision: To be the leading resource for innovative, high-quality and effective health education.

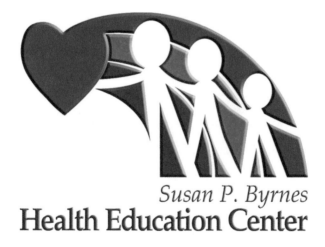

Susan P. Byrnes
Health Education Center

515 South George Street • York, PA 17401
Phone: 717.848.3064 • Toll Free: 800.713.4533
Fax: 717.854.1846
Email: info@byrneshec.com • www.byrneshec.com
www.LearntobeHealthy.org

www.LearntobeHealthy.org

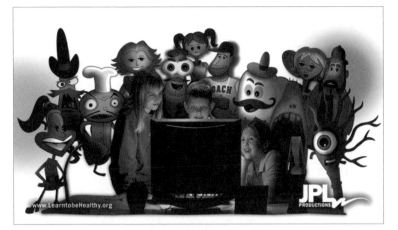

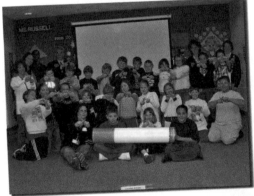

Congressman Todd Platts volunteered to help students at Hanover Middle School learn about the effects of substances on the human body.

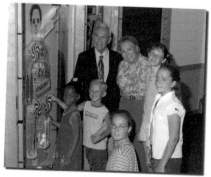

Nancy and Paul Keiser with enthusiastic students.

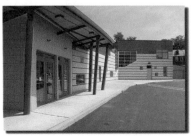

Our bright red doors.

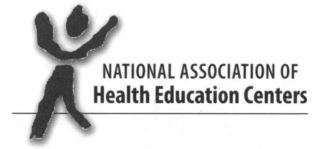

NATIONAL ASSOCIATION OF Health Education Centers

The National Association of Health Education Centers, NAHEC

FACT SHEET

Reaching out to children, families and their health educators

Over 3.7 million children and the adults who care for them are served each year by NAHEC's network of 40 member interactive health education centers and 22 sustaining members in 27 states and the District of Columbia. They serve a vital role in education, especially in improving the well being of the nation's youth, by providing the knowledge and awareness needed to make healthy life decisions, prevent disease and injury, and understand their bodies.

Our Mission and Vision

The mission of NAHEC is to promote the development and advancement of interactive health education centers with the vision to provide all children and the adults who care for them to have access to these programs and resources.

Executive Director: David Midland
1533 W. River Center Dr. • Milwaukee, WI 53212
Phone: 414-390-2188
Fax: 414-390-2199
Email: dmidland@nahec.org

Partners

FULL AFFILIATE AND ASSOCIATE MEMBERS OF NAHEC

Adventure Science Center
Nashville, TN
www.adventuresci.com

Alice Aycock Poe Center for Health Education
Raleigh, NC
www.poehealth.org

CDC Global Health Odyssey
Atlanta, GA
www.cdc.gov/global

Children's Health Education Center
Milwaukee, WI
www.chechealthykids.org

Children's Hospital
Columbus, OH
www.columbuschildrens.com

Clarion University Health Science Education Center
Clarion, PA
www.clarion.edu/hsec

Denver Museum of Nature and Science
Denver, CO
www.dmns.org

Discover Health! Adventures in Learning
Cincinnati, OH
www.discoverhealthnow.org

East Tennessee Discovery Center
Knoxville, TN
www.etdiscovery.org

Elmhurst Memorial Healthcare
Elmhurst, IL
www.emhc.org

Hall of Health
Berkeley, CA
www.hallofhealth.org

Harold W. McMillen Center for Health Education, Inc.
Fort Wayne, IN
www.mcmillencenter.org

The Health Adventure
Asheville, NC
www.thehealthadventure.org

Health Awareness Center
Freehold, NJ
www.centrastate.com

Health Exploration Station
Canton, MI
www.healthexplorationstation.com

Health World
Barrington, IL
www.healthworldmuseum.org

Health World
Scottsdale, AZ
www.healthworldmuseum.org

HealthSpace Cleveland
Cleveland, OH
www.healthspacecleveland.org

HealthWorks! Kids' Museum
South Bend, IN
www.qualityoflife.org/healthworks.htm

Hult Health Education Center
Peoria, IL
www.hult-health.org

John P. McGovern Museum of Health and Medical Science
Houston, TX
www.museumofhealth.org

Kansas Learning Center For Health
Halstead, KS
www.learningcenter.org

HealthMPowers
Atlanta, GA
www.healthmpowers.org

Kleist Health Education Center
Fort Myers, FL
www.fgcu.edu/khec

Lankenau Hospital Health Education Center
Wynnewood, PA
www.mlhs.org

Logansport Health Education Center
Logansport, IN

The Louisville Science Center
Louisville, KY
www.louisvillescience.org

Mercy Health Plan
Chesterfield, MO
www.mercyhealthplans.com

Millis Regional Health Education Center
High Point, NC
www.millishealth.com

MORE HEALTH, Inc.
Tampa, FL
www.morehealthinc.org

National Health Museum
Washington, DC
www.nationalhealthmuseum.org

Robert Crown Center for Health Education
Hinsdale, IL
www.health-ed.org

Roper Mountain Science Center
Greenville, SC
www.ropermountain.org

Ruth Lilly Health Education Center
Indianapolis, IN
www.rlhec.org

Susan P. Byrnes Health Education Center
York, PA
www.byrneshec.com

Weller Health Education Center
Easton, PA
www.wellercenter.org

Wellness Works/Por Su Salud
Grand Island, NE
www.wellnessworksonline.org

West Texas Health Connection
El Paso, TX

QUICK ORDER FORM

Fax orders: 717-854-1846

Telephone orders: Call 717-848-3064 ask for the Giving Coordinator
Have your credit card ready.

Email your orders: www.byrneshec.com

Postal orders: Susan P. Byrnes Health Education Center
515 South George Street
York, PA 17401
717-848-3064

Please send the following book:

_____

_____

_____

Please send me FREE information on:

___ Speaking/Seminars   ___ The Susan P. Byrnes Health Education Center

___ National Association of Health Education Centers

Sales Tax may apply

Shipping costs will vary

Payment: ___ check   ___ credit card:

___ **Visa**   ___ **MasterCard** ___ **American Express**

Card number: _____

Name on card: _____ **Exp. Date** _____

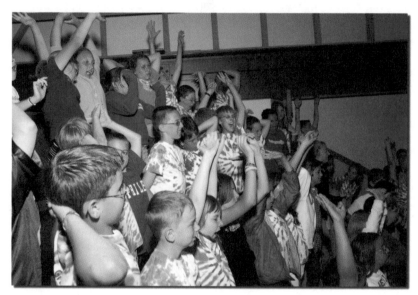

This is all the reward I need ...